Hand of the Wind Taijiquan.
Taoyin Qigong.

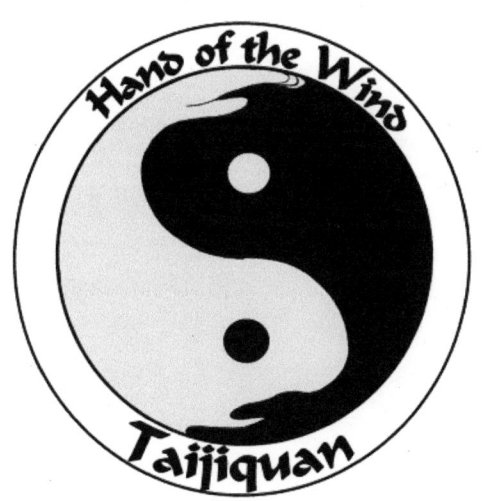

Conrad Robinson

Copyright © 2019 Conrad Robinson. All rights reserved.
Published by Conrad Robinson.
ISBN: 978-0-244-81057-3

Hand of the Wind Taijiquan:

Taoyin Qigong.

Introduction.

Hand of the Wind Taijiquan classes teach the Lee Family Internal Arts which were brought to the U.K. in the first half of the Twentieth Century by Master Chan Kam Lee and then popularized by Master Chee Soo in the second half of the Twentieth Century. The Lee Style is a truly holistic system of Taoist arts which includes the healing arts of Tuina massage, acupuncture, herbal and dietary therapy, heat therapy and Kaimen Taoist Yoga. Alongside the healing arts within the style are the martial arts of Feng Shou Kung Fu, Chin Na and Shuai Jiao. Spanning across both the health and martial aspects of the arts are the Taijiquan (often simply referred to as T'ai Chi) and Qigong.

Qigong simply means to work with Qi, usually translated as 'energy' but more literally translated as 'breath'. However, neither of these translations comes close to providing a true definition of what is meant by Qi. To gain a full understanding of the concept of Qi requires the student to think deeper than the meaning of a single word and consider the ramifications of the term – just as breath indicates life and so much more than just simple inhalation and exhalation. Within a Taoist understanding, Qi makes up the fundamental fabric of the universe. Through practice of Qigong students can develop an awareness of their own Qi and how it affects their health.

Within the Lee style there are several types of Qigong practiced, including:

Standing Qigong (an excellent means of cultivating Qi and developing sensitivity),
Qi Sensitivity Exercises (individual and partnered exercises),
Taiji Qigong (a system of 'Qi balancing' Qigong exercises based upon the movements of the Taiji Form),
Taoyin Qigong (exercises combining movement and breath intended to target specific health benefits).

All of these aspects are taught within Hand of the Wind Taijiquan classes and this book focuses on the Taoyin Qigong system.

Whilst this book does include some basic principles and theory of Qigong training this is not intended to be a book of Qigong theory. Theory is taught within our classes and for those who wish to extend their studies of Qigong theory there are many excellent books on the market already. This book is primarily intended to provide an aide-memoire for Hand of the Wind students to help them remember and practice a variety of Taoyin exercises.

Contents:

Section One:
  Qigong Principles   p7

Section Two:
  Taoyin Qigong Exercises   p16

Section Three:
  Stances   p181

Section Four:
  Index of Taoyin Exercises   p191

Section One:

Qigong Principles.

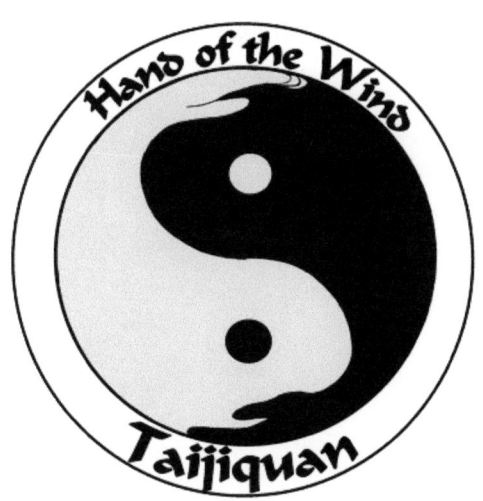

Qigong Principles

When practicing Qigong there are a number of basic principles which we adhere to.
These include:
- Stance and posture,
- Relaxation
- Breathing
- Co-ordination
- Point alignment
- Focus

Within this section, notes are provided to give guidance on how to make these principles a key part of your Qigong practice.

Stance and Posture

Within all of the Lee Family Internal Arts, stance refers to the alignment of the lower body (from the waist down) including weight distribution between the feet. Posture refers to the alignment of the upper body including hand and head positions.

Detailed descriptions of the stances used within the exercises are provided in the third section of this book. Full instruction on the correct application of stance and posture are provided within Hand of the Wind classes.

Key points to remember are:

- Never lock a limb. Knees and elbows are never completely straightened.
- Except where specified in an exercise the head should be aligned naturally with a feeling as if it is suspended from a point just behind the highest point – this extends the neck slightly.
- Shoulders should always be relaxed and 'hang' from the support provided by the natural alignment of the spine.
- Pelvis should be aligned so that the tailbone is tucked underneath the body.
- Weight is supported by the ball of the foot.
- Toes relax onto the floor.
- Stepping into a stance should be heel-toe.
- The tip of the tongue should remain in contact with the roof of the mouth (as if about to make the 'L' sound).

Relaxation

At all times it is important for the body and mind to remain as relaxed as possible. The more tension there is in the body, then the harder it is for Qi to flow. Within each exercise the aim is to use the minimum amount of tension in order to achieve the intended posture.

Breathing

Correct breathing technique is vital to get the full benefits of Qigong practice. Again, the key is relaxation. It is our aim to breathe as deeply as possible whilst maintaining full relaxation. Techniques to increase relaxed breathing capability are taught within Hand of the Wind classes.

As a starting point, aim to be aware of your breathing. Follow the breath down into your body as you inhale and then as soon as you start to feel tension build within the body allow yourself to exhale. Over time you should be able to feel that you can inhale deeper before tension starts to build.

It is tension within the body that inhibits our ability to utilize the full capacity of our lungs. By increasing the relaxation of the intercostal muscles, the diaphragm, the abdominals and the muscles of the back we can allow our lungs to more fully expand. This increases our ability to expel carbon dioxide and draw oxygen into our bodies.

Coordination

During Taoyin exercises the movements are tied to the breath. You should focus on timing the movement to fit with your own breath whilst maintaining relaxation. This is the reason why you will get the most benefits from your practice of Taoyin exercises when you perform them at your own pace, rather than at the 'teaching speed' at which exercises are performed within classes.

It takes practice to be able to properly coordinate the movements of both stance and posture with the breath. Initially, concentrate on learning the movement and then work on coordinating the timing and precision of the movements.

Point Alignment

Within Qigong and Chinese Medical theory, it is understood that Qi naturally follows certain pathways through the body. These pathways are referred to as Channels or Meridians and relate to specific organ functions. There are twelve main channels through the body, six flow along the arms and six flow along the legs. The specific benefits of each Taoyin exercise are linked to how the movements of the exercise encourage Qi to flow along these channels. The specific location of each channel is beyond the remit of this book, but there are many publications available detailing Meridian location for those students who are interested.

Channels are classed as either Yin or Yang depending upon the direction of their Qi flow. Yin channels flow upwards (assuming hands are held above the head) and are primarily located on the front of the body. Yang channels flow downwards and are mostly located on the back of the body. Yin and Yang channels are paired so that the Heart channel (Yin) pairs with the Small Intestine (Yang); Lung (Yin) with Large Intestine; Spleen (Yin) with Stomach; Kidney (Yin) with Bladder; Liver (Yin) with Gall Bladder; Heart Protector (Yin – sometimes referred to as Pericardium) with Triple Heater (Yang).

Along each channel there are points where the Qi can be accessed easily and these are the points used in Acupuncture and Acupressure to treat ailments. Within our Qigong training there are certain points we focus on, where Qi can most freely enter and leave the body and these are referred to as 'Gates'.

As well as the twelve channels relating to organs, there are eight other major Qi pathways through the body. These primarily act as reservoirs of Qi and are often called Special Vessels. They are the Governing Vessel, Conception Vessel, Belt or Girdle Vessel, Penetrating Vessel, Linking Vessels and the Heel Vessels. Within our Qigong practice the Governing, Conception and Belt vessels are the most relevant. The Governing Vessel runs up the centre line of the back of the torso and over the top of the head to the mouth. The Conception vessel runs up the centre line of the front of the torso and to the mouth. The Belt vessel is the only channel that runs horizontally on the body and (with a few kinks along the way!) it passes around the waist.

Whilst performing Qigong exercises it is important to be aware of how you are aligning the 'Gates' within each posture. To this end, brief descriptions of the location of the most important gates are found in the following table. There are numerous good resources for more detailed point location notes on the internet or in the many published books on the subject.

'Gate' location table:

Gate	Location	Channel
Bubbling Spring	On the bottom of the ball of the foot.	Kidney (KD 1)
Lao Gong	In the centre of the palm of the hand.	Heart Protector (HP 8)
He Gu	On the bulge of muscle between the base of the thumb and the forefinger.	Large Intestine (LI 4)
Qi Hu	On the front of the body, just below the centre of the clavicle.	Stomach (ST 13)
Yang Gu	The little finger edge of the wrist.	Small Intestine (SI 5)
Huan Tiao	On the side of the buttock, where the gluteus maximus muscle meets the hip joint.	Gall Bladder (GB 30)
Lower Tantien	On the centre line of the front of the body, 2 inches below the navel.	Conception Vessel (CV 4)
Middle Tantien	On the centre line of the front of the body, in the mid-point of the sternum.	Conception Vessel (CV 17)
Upper Tantien	On the centre line of the front of the forehead, the 'third eye' point.	Governor Vessel (Not a numbered point)
Bai Hui	On the top of the head, on the centre line.	Governor Vessel (GV 20)
Hui Yin	On the centre line, half-way between the genitals and anus.	Conception Vessel (CV 1)

Focus

Taoyin exercises are often referred to as 'Guide and Stretch' exercises. We guide the Qi with our minds as we stretch the body. Focusing the mind on the desired flow of Qi will strengthen the effects of the exercises and improve the health benefits of each exercise.

Initially, it is important to develop sensitivity to Qi whilst performing the exercises. Relax the mind and aim to feel any sensations throughout the body. As you feel more happening within your body during the exercises, you will increase your awareness of Qi and this will inform your ability to direct your Qi correctly within the exercises.

Section Two:

Taoyin Qigong Exercises.

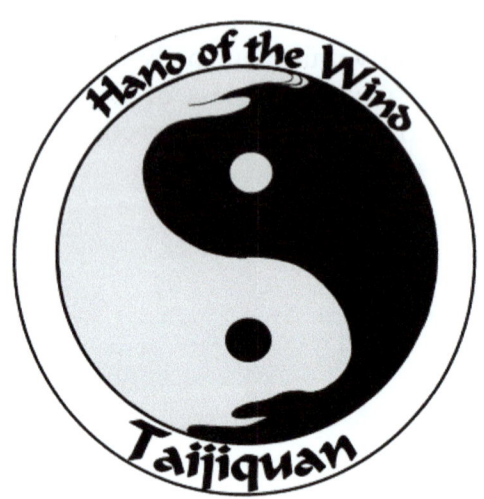

Taoyin Qigong Exercises.

What follows is a small selection of the Taoyin Qigong exercises taught within the Lee Family Internal Arts; the specific exercises presented in this book are some of the most commonly taught within Hand of the Wind classes. The exercises are described in terms of stance and posture movements to be performed whilst breathing in or out as shown in the description. Remember to time the movement to your breath.

The exercises are presented in alphabetical order to make it easier for the reader to find a specific exercise to practice. The descriptions indicate which organ systems or channels each exercise targets, although this is only intended to give a general idea – it is important to consult a qualified and experienced instructor to determine which exercises would be most beneficial for you and for specific ailments. Some exercises are listed as 'balancing' exercises and these are exercises that help to balance the Qi throughout the whole body and therefore can be said to benefit all of the organs.

Normally, each exercise should be repeated four or eight times.

The exercises shown in this book are just a small selection from the much greater number of exercises contained within the Lee Family system of Taoyin Qigong. It is strongly recommended that students continue to maintain their own notes on exercises taught within classes to expand their repertoire of available Taoyin.

Notes on the illustrations accompanying each exercise description:

Each exercise description is accompanied by photographs of the end point of each movement (corresponding with the end of each 'in' or 'out' breath). The image is taken from the 'front' of the room in each case. Where there are multiple photographs the following guidelines apply:

Photographs of the same height show the end points of the movement and show the position from the front and side viewpoints.

Smaller images show 'transitional' points within the movement and progress from left to right as the movement progresses. These are intended to help the reader perform the movements accurately and clarify aspects where there could be confusion.

Remember that posture and stance movements should be synchronized with each other and with the breath during all exercises.

The Archer Turns Around

Benefits: Lungs and Heart.

Start Position:

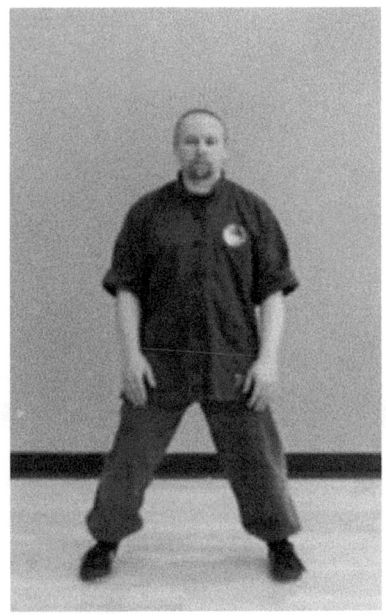

Stance: Remain in Riding Horse stance throughout the exercise.
Posture: Arms relaxed at sides, head neutral.

The Archer Turns Around (continued)

Breathing In:

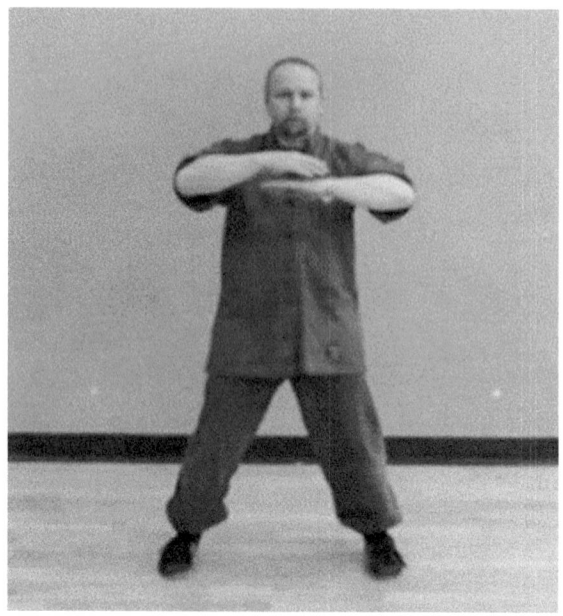

Posture: The hands come up in front of the centre line of the body, with the palms facing downwards, until they are at chest height. Right hand above left.

The Archer Turns Around (continued)

Breathing Out:

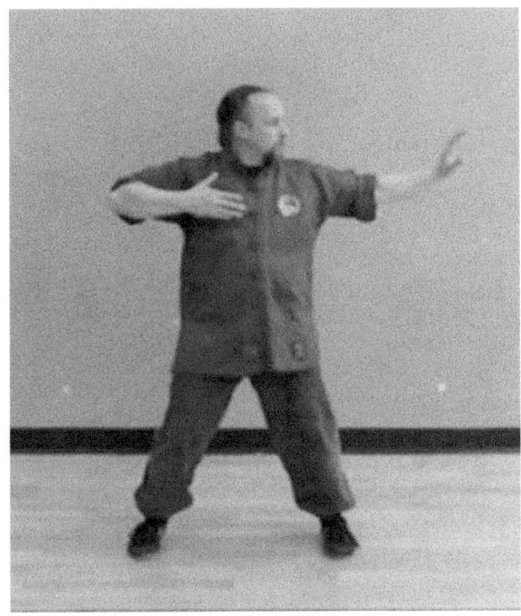

Posture: The left hand moves out to the left side of the body with the palm facing away from the body. The head turns to follow as the eyes watch the left hand. The right hand turns to face the palm towards the body and the elbow 'pulls' away to the right, drawing the hand to in front of the shoulder (Lao Gong towards Qi Hu).

The Archer Turns Around (continued)

Breathing In:

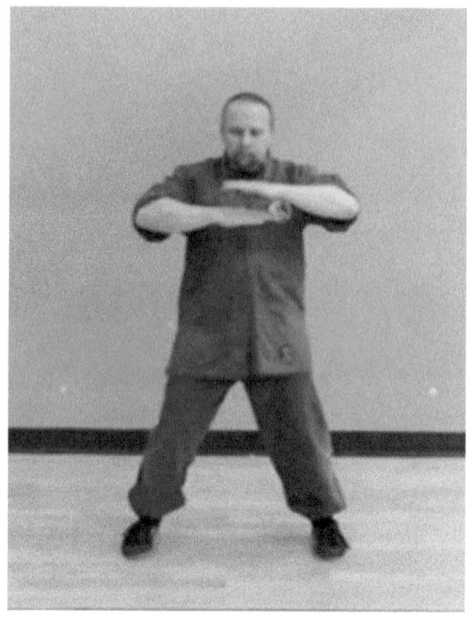

Posture: The hands return to in front of the chest with the palms down. This time with the left hand above the right.

The Archer Turns Around (continued)

Breathing Out:

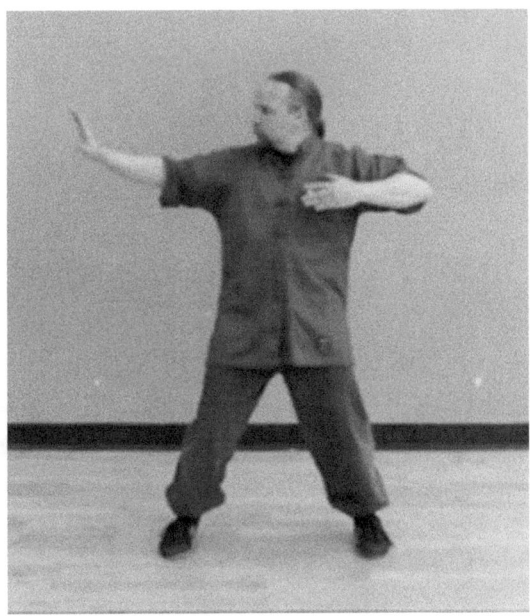

Posture: The right hand moves out to the right side of the body with the palm facing away from the body. The head turns to follow as the eyes watch the right hand. The left hand turns to face the palm towards the body and the elbow 'pulls' away to the left, drawing the hand to in front of the shoulder.

The Archer Turns Around (continued)

Breathing In:

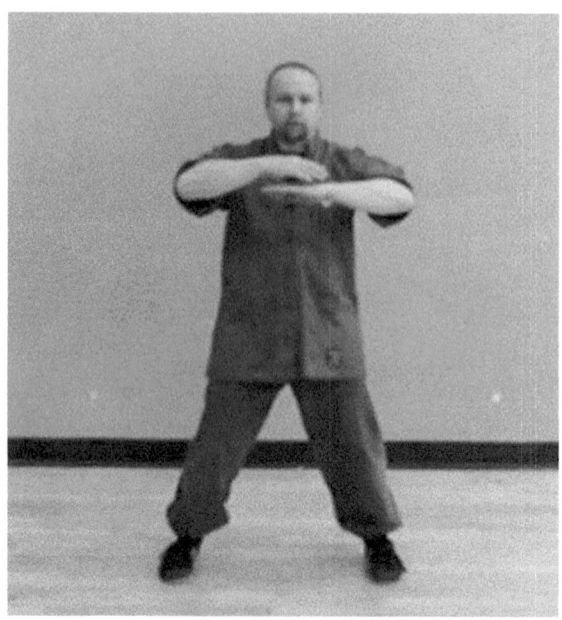

Posture: The hands return to in front of the chest with the palms down. This time with the right hand above the left.

Notes: Continue the pattern to repeat the exercise 4 or 8 times on each side. On the 'Out' breath, ensure that the hand 'pushing' out to the side and being watched comes out from underneath the other hand and then returns to the 'top' position on the 'In' breath.

The Archer Turns Around (continued)

Breathing Out:

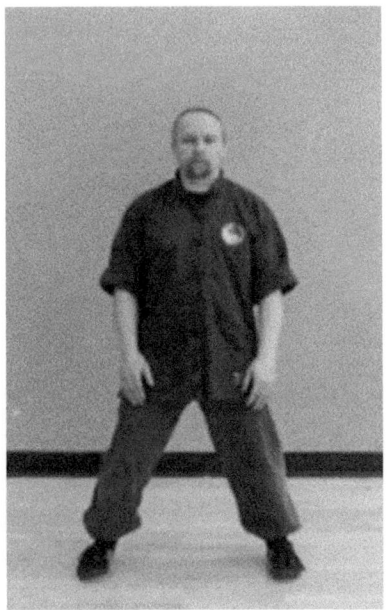

Posture: From the final 'In' breath position (hands palms down in front of chest with right hand above left) the hands lower down in front of the centre line to finish in relaxed position by the sides.

Bend and Twist

Benefits: Kidney, Liver and Spleen.

Start Position:

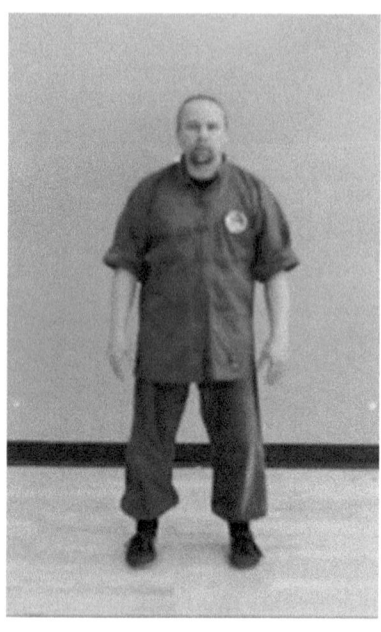

Stance: Remain in Bear stance throughout this exercise.
Posture: Arms relaxed at sides, head in neutral position.

Bend and Twist (continued)

Breathing In:

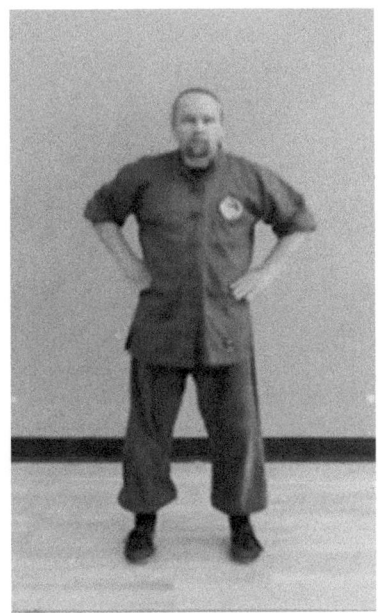

Posture: Hands come up to rest on the waist, palms down with the thumbs behind the body and fingers to the front – this connects the He Gu point with the Belt vessel.

Bend and Twist (continued)

Breathing Out:

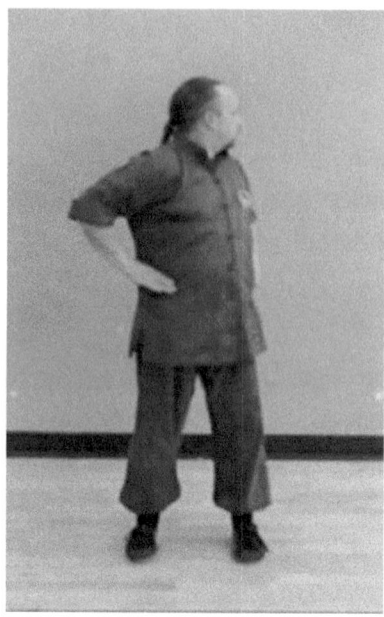

Posture: Keeping the hands in position, turn the body (from the waist) towards your left – aim to maintain the Bear stance so that the hips continue to face the front.

Bend and Twist (continued)

Breathing In:

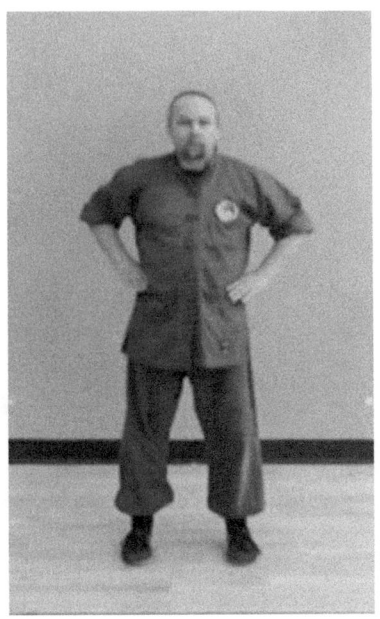

Posture: Hands stay on waist, straighten the body back to face the front.

Bend and Twist (continued)

Breathing Out:

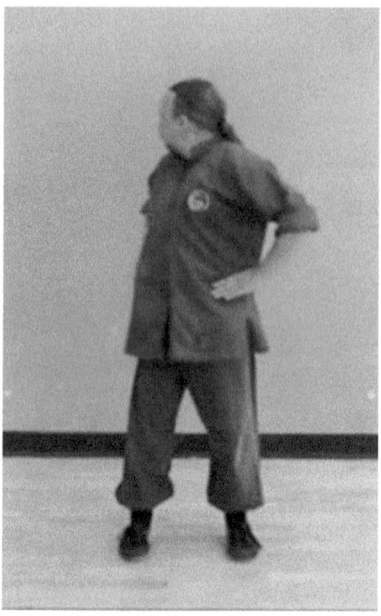

Posture: Keeping the hands in position, turn the body (from the waist) towards your right – again, aim to maintain the Bear stance so that the hips continue to face the front.

Bend and Twist (continued)

Breathing In:

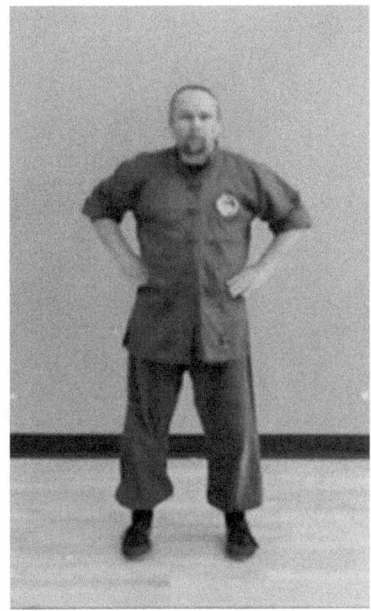

Posture: Hands stay on waist, straighten the body back to face the front.

Bend and Twist (continued)

Breathing Out:

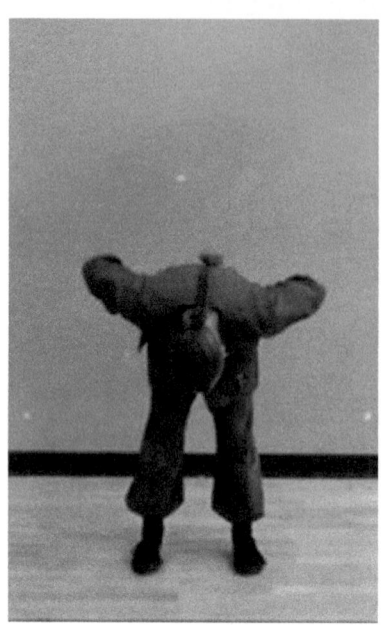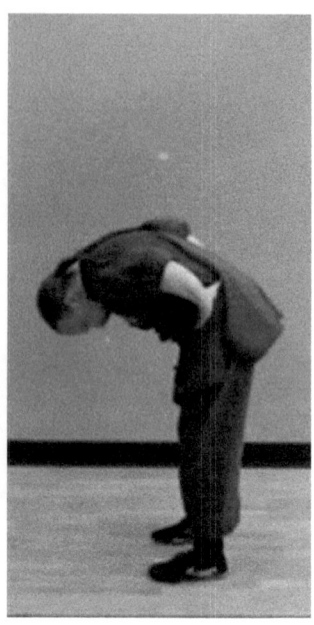

Posture: Still keeping the hands on the waist, lean forwards (from the waist) and then bring the chin towards the chest.

Bend and Twist (continued)

Breathing In:

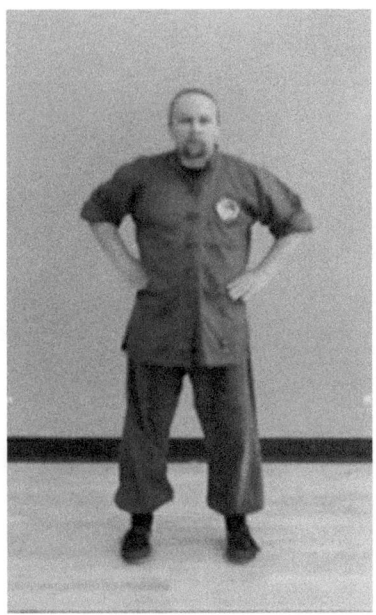

Posture: Bring the head back into neutral position with the neck and then straighten the body carefully (again from the waist).

Bend and Twist (continued)

Breathing Out:

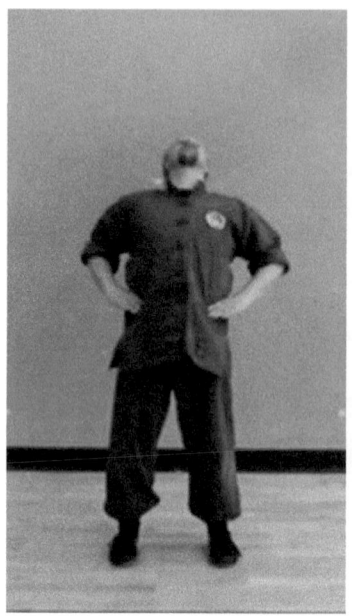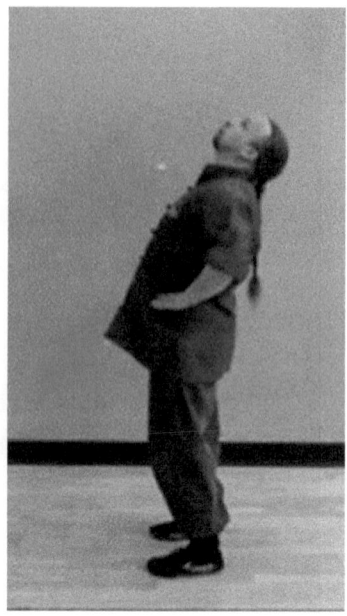

Posture: Hands remain on waist. Carefully (without over-stretching) lean the body backwards from the waist. At the end of the movement raise the chin away from the chest – be careful not to compress the back of the neck but to open the front of the neck upwards.

Bend and Twist (continued)

Breathing In:

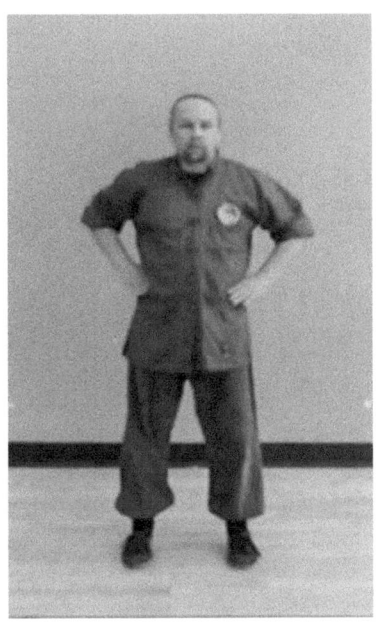

Posture: Bring the head back into neutral position with the neck and then straighten the body carefully (again from the waist).

Bend and Twist (continued)

Breathing Out:

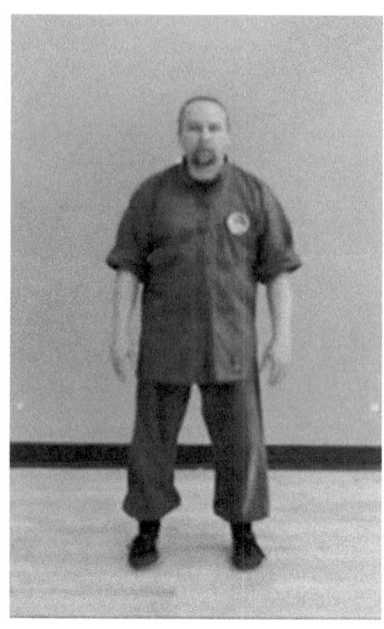

Posture: Lower the hands to the sides into neutral position.

Notes: Be careful not to over-stretch during this exercise – if you twist or bend too far, you are likely to only notice it as you straighten - at which point you may have already pulled a muscle!

Repeat the exercise 4 or 8 times.

The Dragon Spits Fire

Benefits: Liver and Spleen.

Start Position:

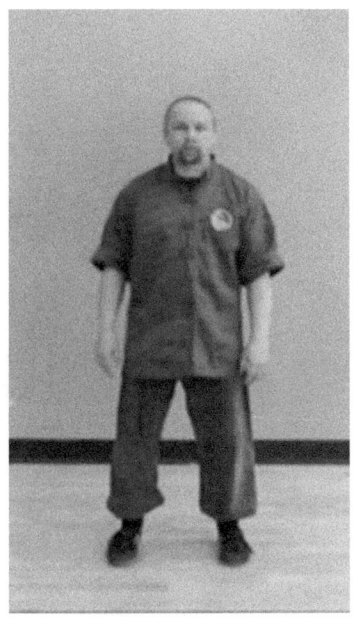

Stance: Start in Bear stance.
Posture: Arms relaxed at sides, head in neutral position.

The Dragon Spits Fire (continued)

Breathing In:

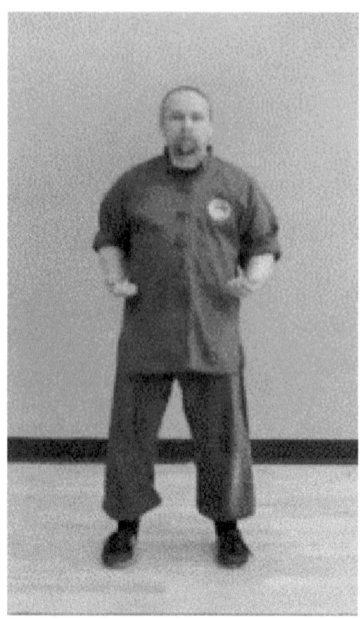

Stance: Remain in Bear stance.
Posture: The hands come up to waist height, palms upwards in 'loose' fists.

The Dragon Spits Fire (continued)

Breathing Out:

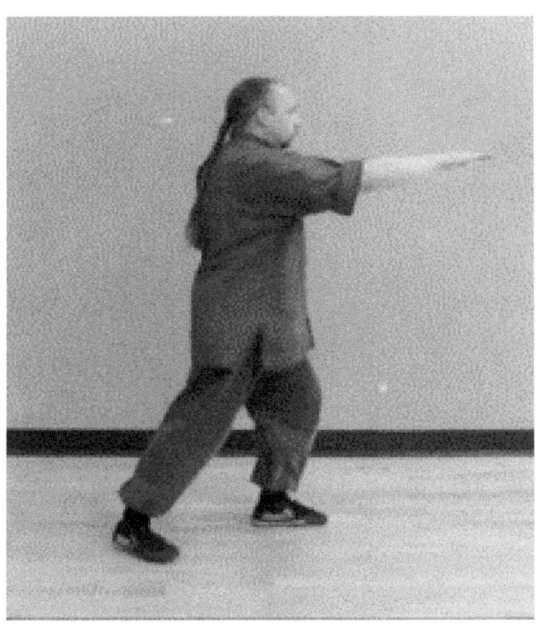

Stance: Step the left foot off to the left to come into a Left Dragon stance facing to your left, correcting the right foot as the weight settles into the Dragon. Ensure that you are in a correct Dragon with the feet shoulder width apart, so that you are not 'walking a tightrope' with one foot directly in front of the other.
Posture: The right hand opens and turns palm downwards as it extends out to in front of the right shoulder (shoulder height, extended forwards).

The Dragon Spits Fire (continued)

Breathing In:

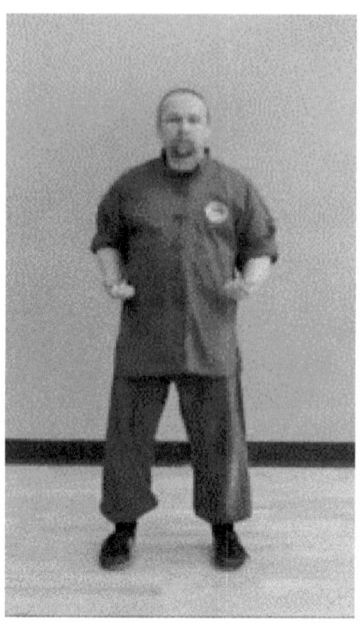

Stance: Correct the right foot and then transition the weight onto it before stepping the left foot back into a Bear stance facing the front as at the start of the exercise.
Posture: The right hand returns to a soft fist, palm up at waist height next to the body.

The Dragon Spits Fire (continued)

Breathing Out:

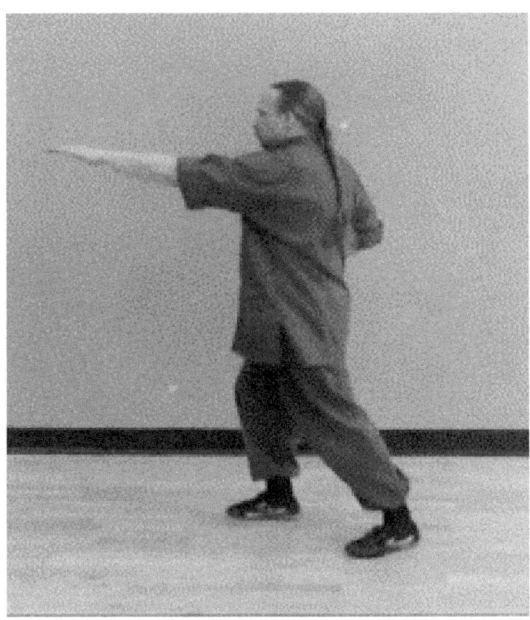

Stance: As in the previous out breath but this time stepping the right foot to finish in a Right Dragon stance facing to the right.

Posture: Again, as in the previous out breath but this time extending the right hand forwards, palm down.

The Dragon Spits Fire (continued)

Breathing In:

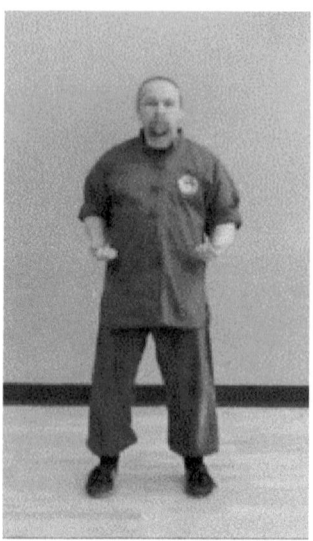

Stance: Return to Bear stance facing the front again as in the original start position.

Posture: The left hand returns to a soft fist, palm up at waist height beside the body.

Notes: Continue the pattern, alternating stepping to the right and left into Dragon stances and extending the corresponding hand. On the 'in' breaths, return to Bear stance facing the 'front' (the original direction you faced at the start of the exercise). Aim to step 4 or 8 times to each side.

The Dragon Spits Fire (continued)

Breathing Out:

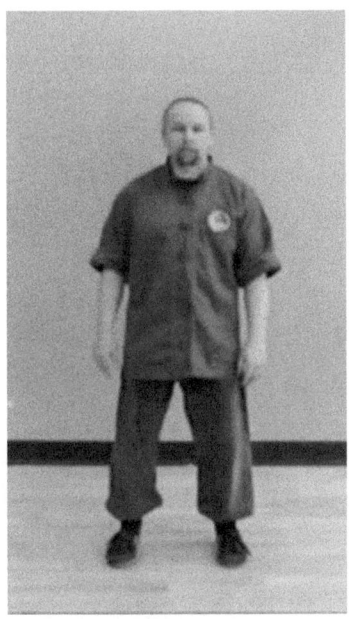

Stance: Remain in Bear stance.
Posture: Hands open and lower down to the sides.

Notes: As you perform the exercise, be aware of the twisting or spiraling motion of the hand as it moves to and from the fist to the palm down and extended position.

Expand the Chest

Benefits: Lungs

Start Position:

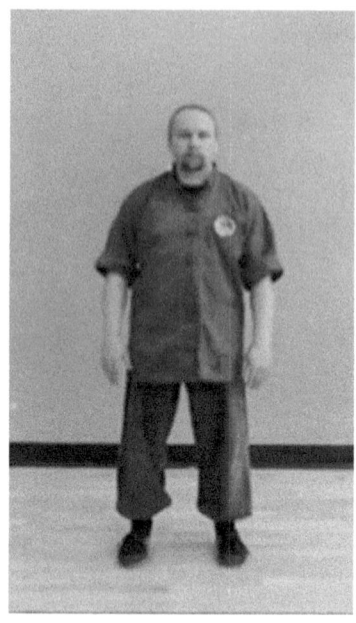

Stance: Remain in Bear stance throughout this exercise.
Posture: Arms relaxed at sides, head in neutral position.

Expand the Chest (continued)

Breathing In:

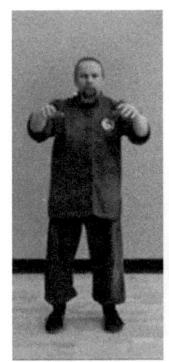 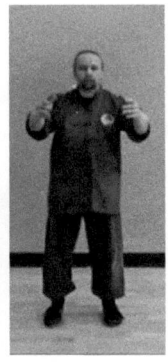 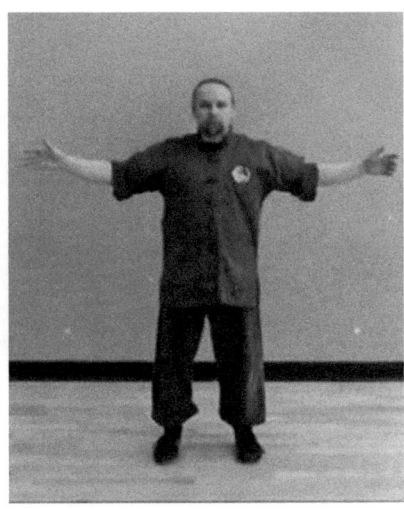

Posture: Hands raise up in front of body with the palms facing downwards until the hands are at chest height. The hands then turn so that the palms are facing each other and then move out to the sides, remaining at chest height.

Expand the Chest (continued)

Breathing Out:

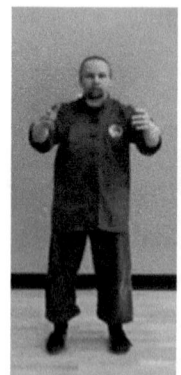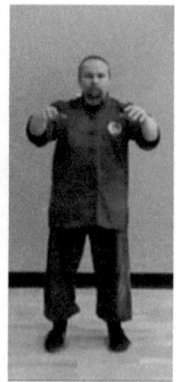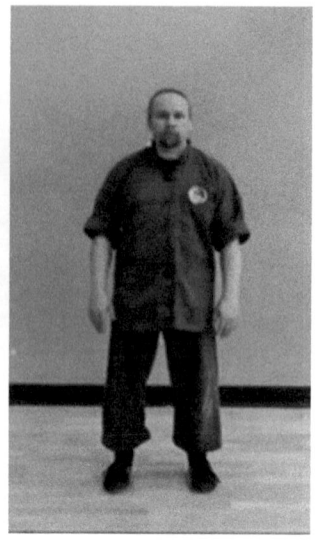

Posture: The hands come back in until they are in front of the body, still at chest height so that the palms face each other. Then the hands turn so that the palms face downwards and the hands then lower to the start position with arms by sides.

Notes: Repeat the in and out breaths until you have completed 8 repetitions. When opening the arms out to the sides, be aware of the expansion of the chest.

The Flying Fox

Benefits: Lungs and Kidneys.

Start Position:

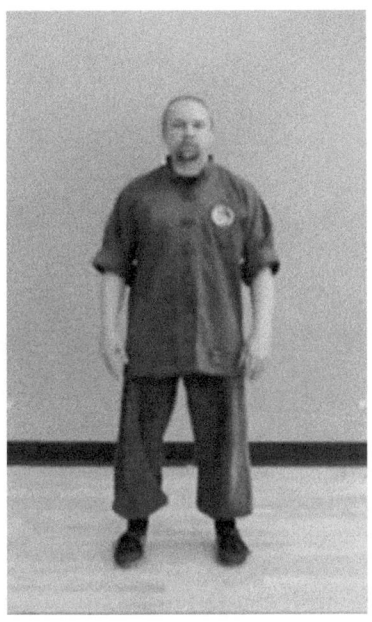

Stance: Remain in Bear stance throughout this exercise.
Posture: Arms relaxed at sides, head in neutral position.

The Flying Fox (continued)

Breathing In:

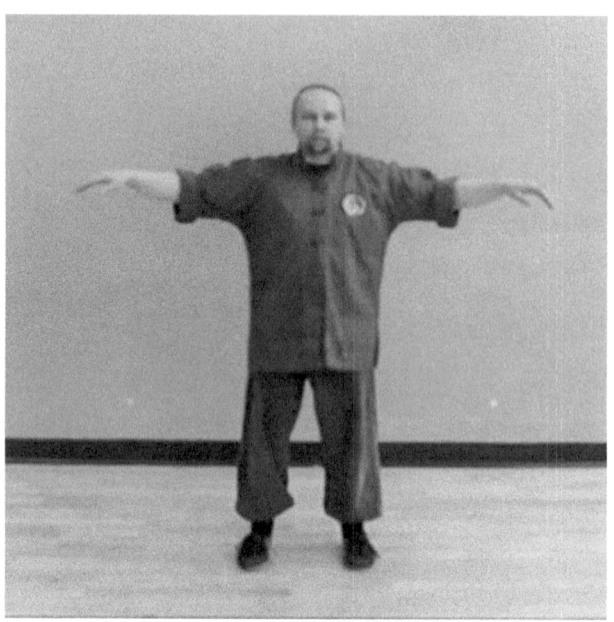

Posture: Hands rise up and out to sides to finish at shoulder height, extended to sides with palms down.

The Flying Fox (continued)

Breathing Out:

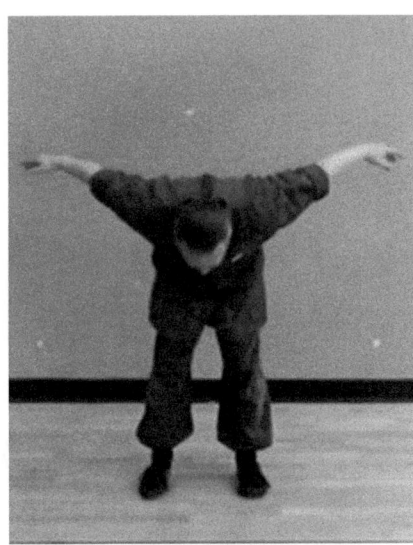
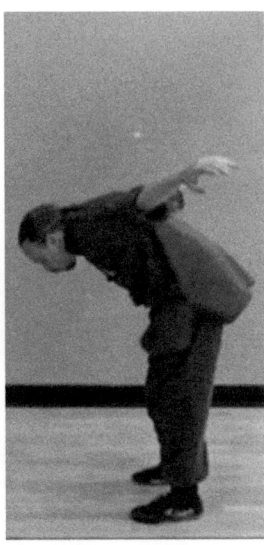

Posture: Maintaining the Bear stance, lean forwards from the waist keeping the hands at the original shoulder height (this means the arms will need to extend up and backwards as the body leans forwards).

The Flying Fox (continued)

Breathing In:

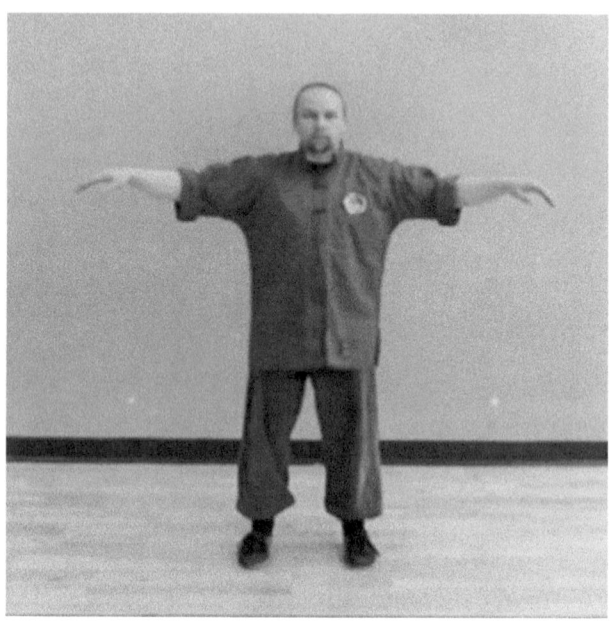

Posture: Straighten the body back with the arms maintaining the same height extended to sides – as you bring the body up 'push' away from the body with the fingertips.

Notes: Repeat the out and in breaths, leaning forwards and straightening up until you have done 8 repetitions.

The Flying Fox (continued)

Breathing Out:

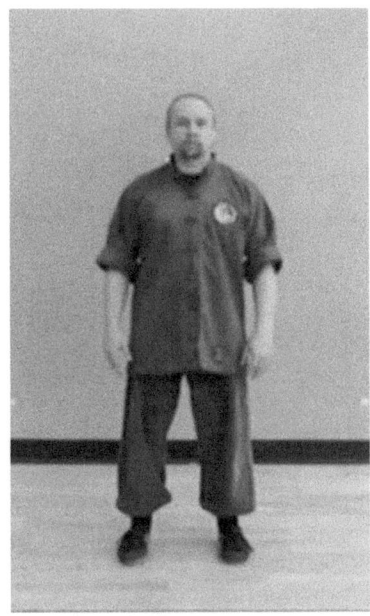

Posture: Lower arms back down to the sides.

Notes: When straightening back up on the in breaths it is important to extend the fingers away from the body to the sides as the body lifts – this releases tension from the shoulders.

Fly like the Dove

Benefits: Lungs.

Start Position:

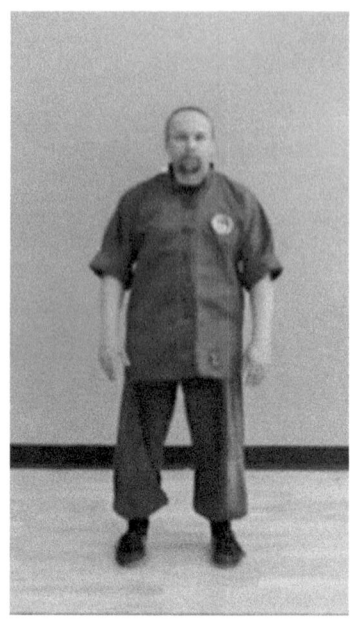

Stance: Remain in Bear stance throughout this exercise.
Posture: Arms relaxed at sides, head in neutral position.

Fly like the Dove (continued)

Breathing In:

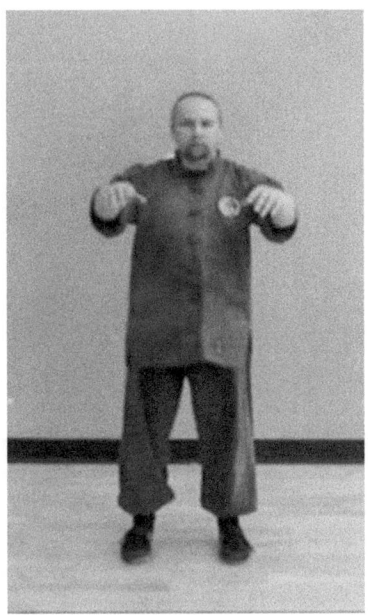

Posture: Hands raise up in front of body with the palms facing downwards until the hands are at chest height.

Fly like the Dove (continued)

Breathing Out:

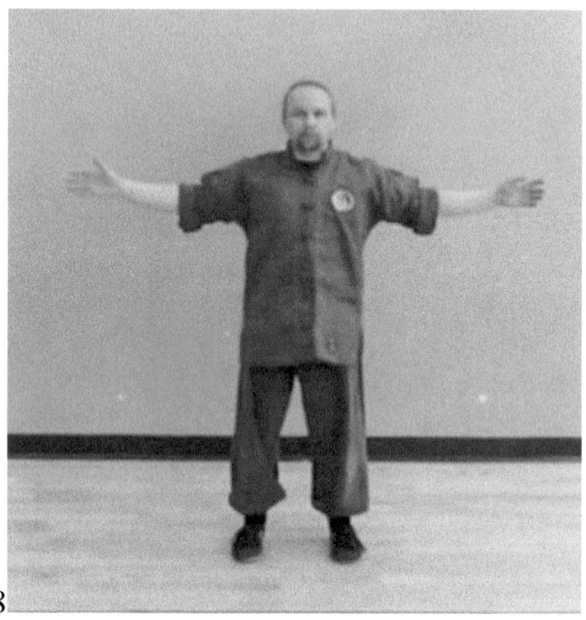

8

Posture: The hands turn so that the palms are facing each other and then move out to the sides, remaining at chest height.

Fly like the Dove (continued)

Breathing In:

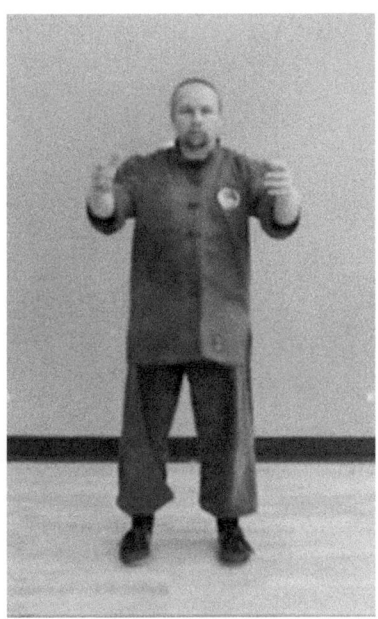

Posture: The hands come back in until they are in front of the body, still at chest height so that the palms face each other.

Notes: Repeat the out and in breaths, opening the hands outwards and then returning to in front of chest, until you have completed 8 repetitions.

Fly like the Dove (continued)

Breathing Out:

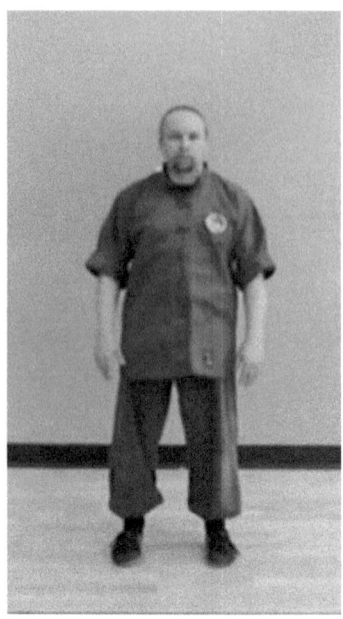

Posture: The hands turn so that the palms face downwards and the hands then lower to the start position with arms by sides.

Notes: When opening the arms out to the sides, be aware of the expansion of the chest.

Fly like the Wild Goose

Benefits: Heart.

Start Position:

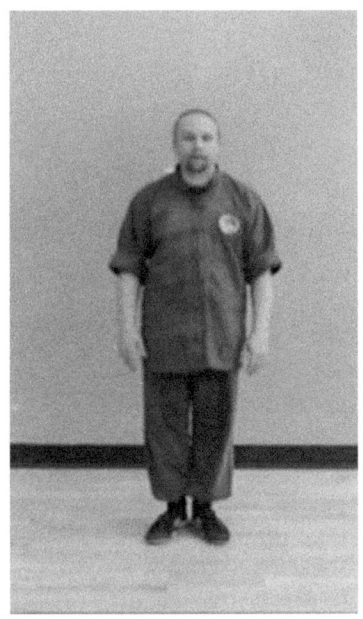

Stance: Begin in Eagle stance.
Posture: Arms relaxed by sides, head neutral.

Fly like the Wild Goose (continued)

Breathing In:

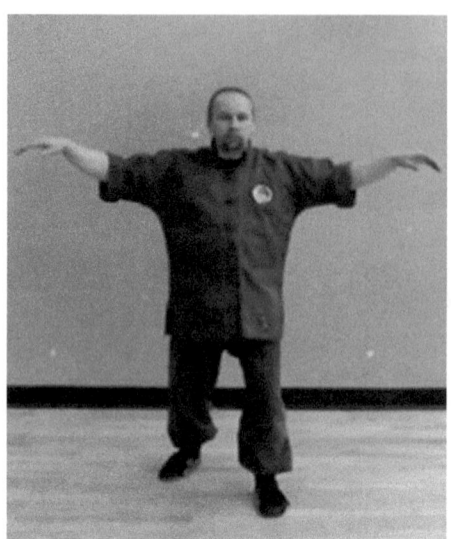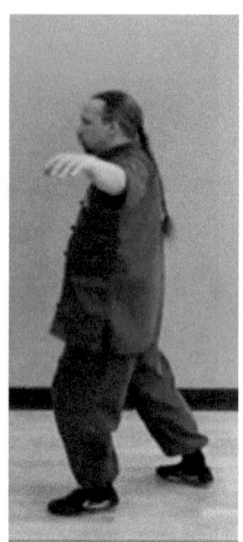

Stance: Step the left foot forwards into position to then be able to bring the weight forwards into Dragon stance.
Posture: Arms both rise up and out to sides with palms down until at shoulder height.

Fly like the Wild Goose (continued)

Breathing Out:

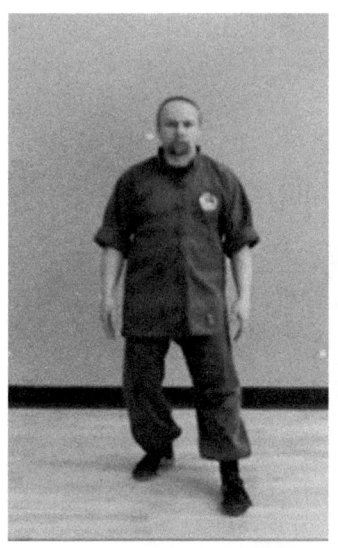 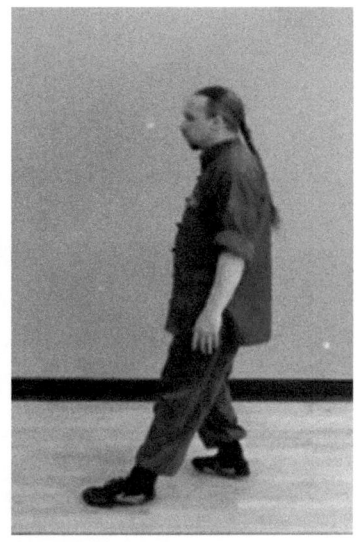

Stance: Draw the weight back into a Duck stance.
Posture: Arms lower to neutral position by the sides.

Notes: Repeat in and out breaths 'rocking' between Left Dragon and Left Duck until you have come forwards into the Dragon 4 or 8 times.

Fly like the Wild Goose (continued)

Breathing Out:

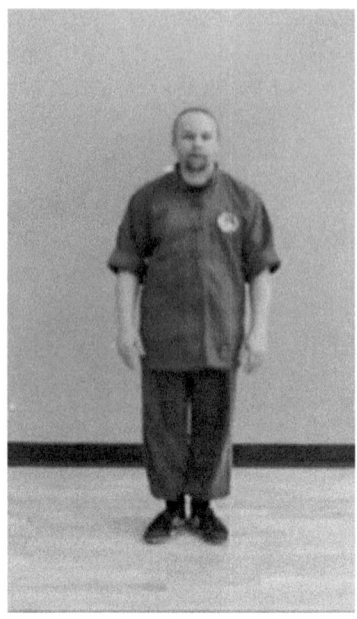

Stance: Draw the weight back into a Duck stance and then bring the left foot back into an Eagle stance.
Posture: Arms lower to neutral position by the sides.

Fly like the Wild Goose (continued)

Breathing In:

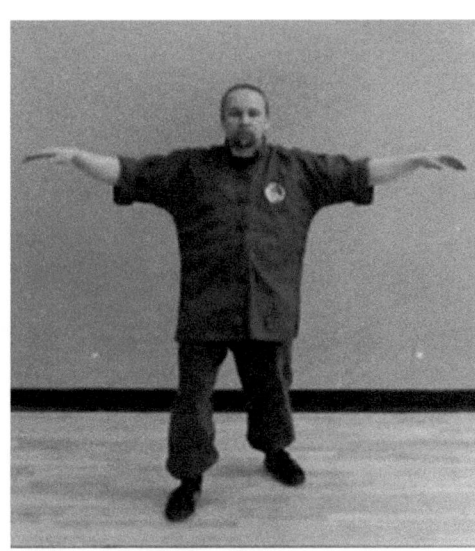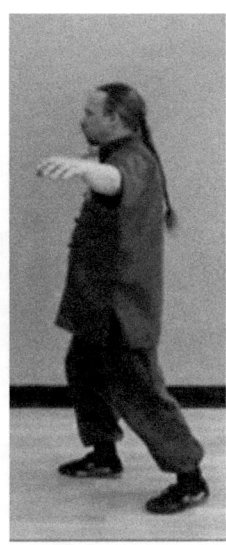

Stance: Step the Right foot forwards into position to then be able to bring the weight forwards into Dragon stance.

Posture: Arms both rise up and out to sides with palms down until at shoulder height.

Fly like the Wild Goose (continued)

Breathing Out:

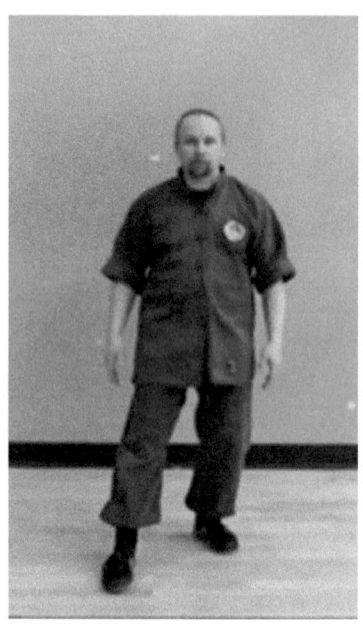 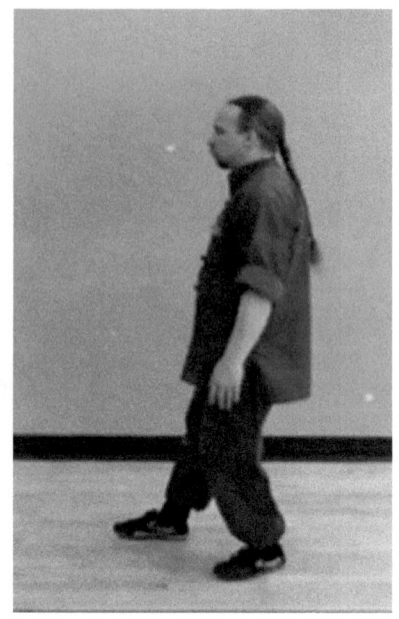

Stance: Draw the weight back into a Duck stance.
Posture: Arms lower to neutral position by the sides.

Notes: Repeat in and out breaths 'rocking' between Right Dragon and Right Duck until you have come forwards into the Dragon 4 or 8 times.

Fly like the Wild Goose (continued)

Breathing Out:

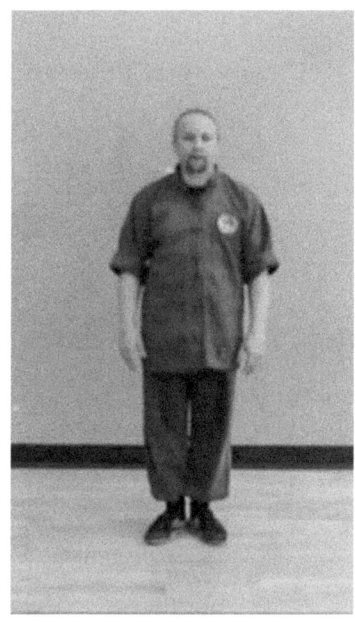

Stance: Draw the weight back into a Duck stance and then bring the left foot back into an Eagle stance.
Posture: Arms lower to neutral position by the sides.

Notes: This exercise can also be performed as a 'static' exercise rather than the 'rocking' exercise as described above – simply remain in Bear stance as you synchronize the arm movements and breath.

Four Directional Breathing

Benefits: Balancing Qigong

Start Position:

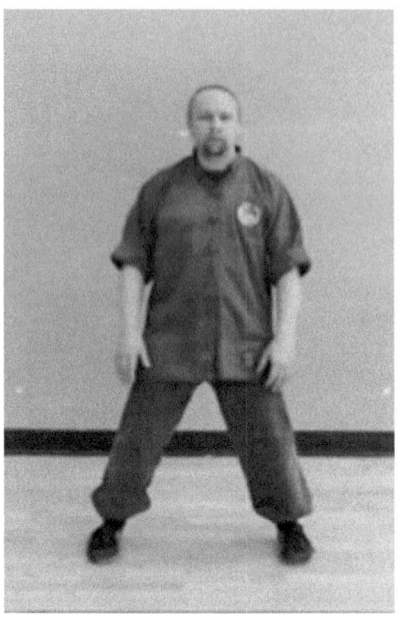

Stance: Remain in Riding Horse stance throughout the exercise.
Posture: Arms relaxed at sides, head neutral.

Four Directional Breathing (continued)

Breathing In:

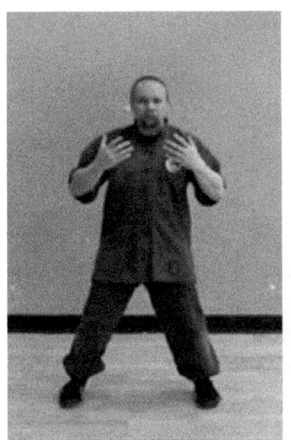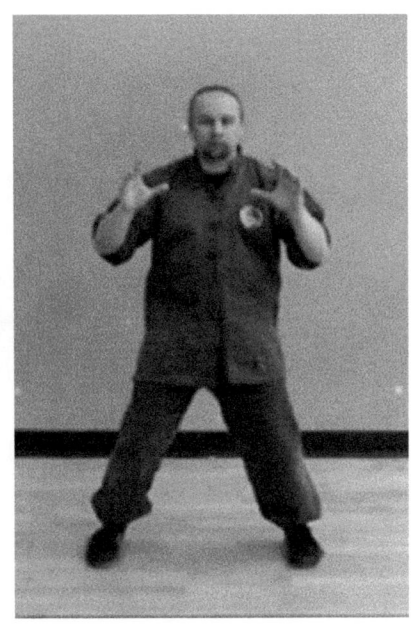

Posture: Hands come up in front of body, palms facing in towards body until hands are in front of shoulders with fingers pointing upwards. The hands then turn (as if around two 'balls') until the back of the hands are facing the body.

Four Directional Breathing (continued)

Breathing Out:

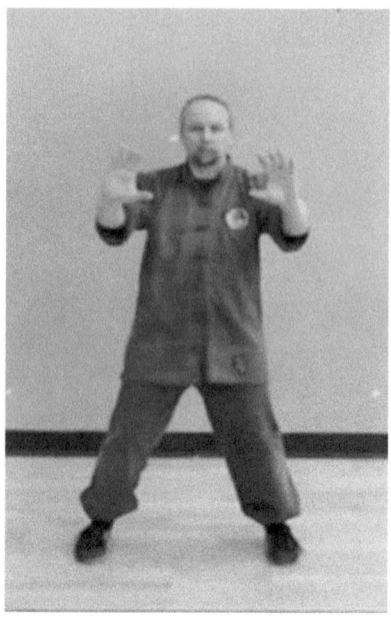

Posture: The hands 'push' forwards to an extended position at shoulder height.

Four Directional Breathing (continued)

Breathing In:

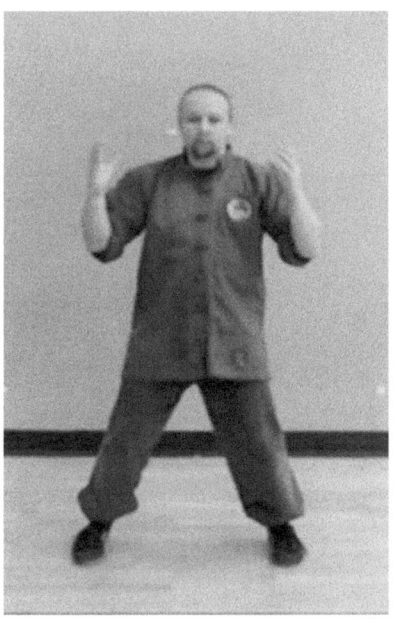

Posture: The hands turn to palms inwards and return towards the shoulders before again circling around two 'balls' until palms are facing each other.

Four Directional Breathing (continued)

Breathing Out:

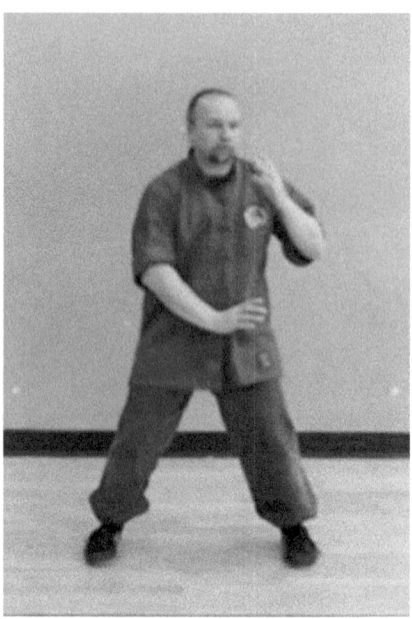

Posture: The right hand 'pushes' down and across the front of the body diagonally until it is in front of the left hip.

Four Directional Breathing (continued)

Breathing in:

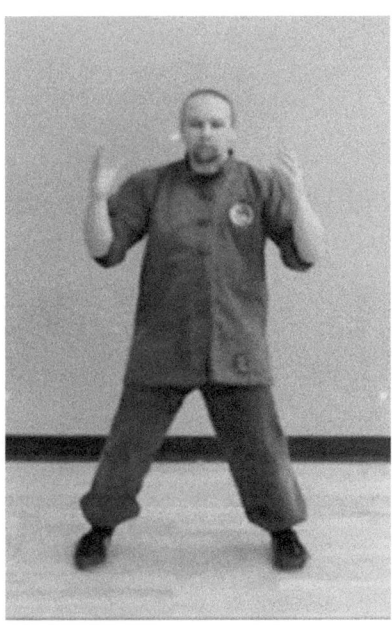

Posture: The right hand turns palm inwards and returns to in front of the right shoulder. Both hands then circle around two 'balls' until palms are facing each other again.

Four Directional Breathing (continued)

Breathing Out:

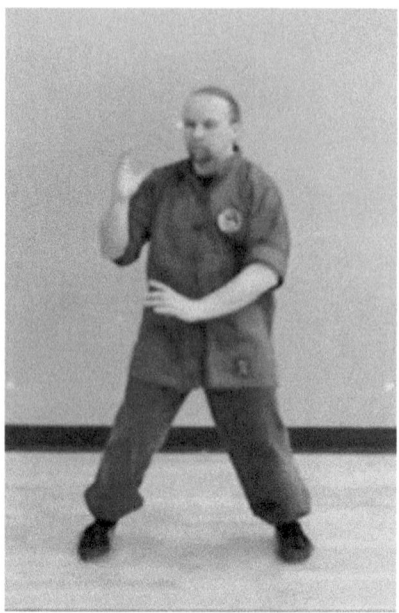

Posture: The left hand 'pushes' down and across the front of the body diagonally to in front of the right hip.

Four Directional Breathing (continued)

Breathing In:

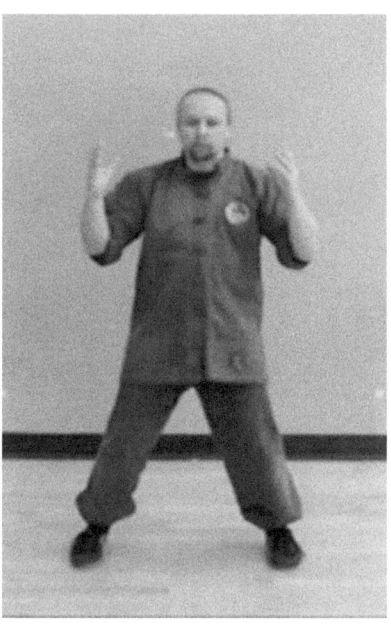

Posture: The left hand turns palm inwards and returns to in front of left shoulder. Both hands then circle around two 'balls' until palms are facing each other again.

Four Directional Breathing (continued)

Breathing Out:

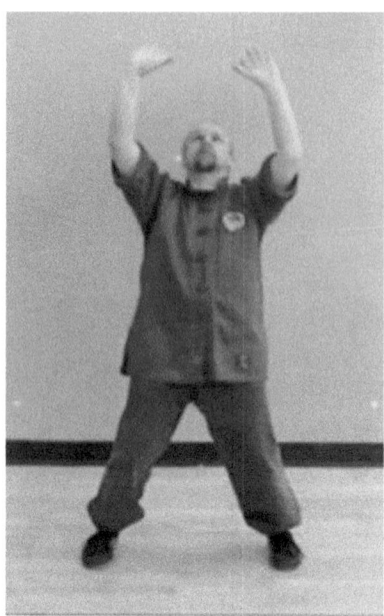

Posture: Both hands turn to palms upwards and push up above head. The head follows the hands to look upwards.

Four Directional Breathing (continued)

Breathing in:

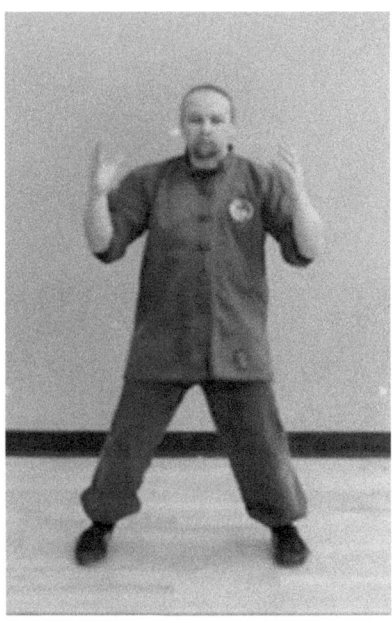

Posture: Hands turn inwards and return to in front of the shoulders and then circle to face each other. Head returns to neutral as the hands come downwards.

Four Directional Breathing (continued)

Breathing In:

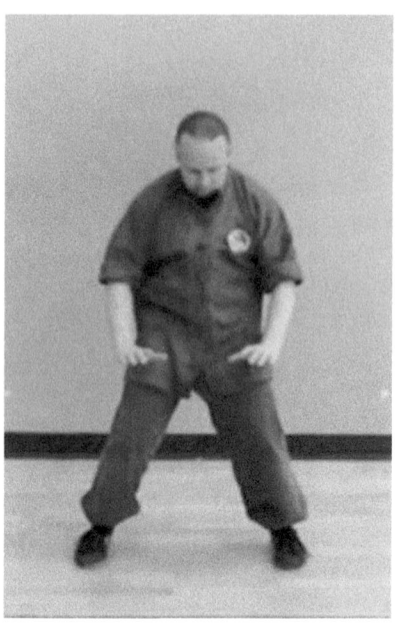

Posture: Both hands turn to palms down and press down in front of the body, until lower than the navel. The head once again follows the hand movement to look downwards.

Four Directional Breathing (continued)

Breathing In:

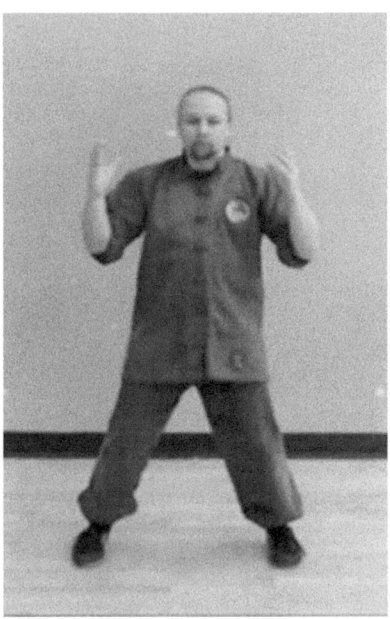

Posture: The hands turn palm inwards and return to in front of the shoulders and then circle to palms facing each other.

Four Directional Breathing (continued)

Breathing Out:

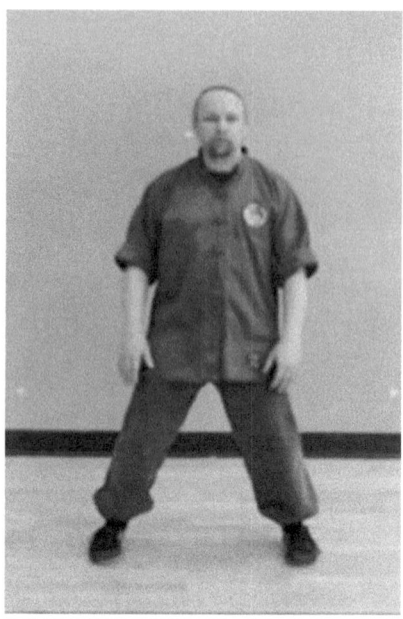

Posture: The hands lower down to neutral position by the sides.

Notes: This is the exercise that we use as part of the warm-up at Hand of the Wind Taijiquan classes. It is a good exercise for opening up all of the channels and encouraging Qi to flow throughout the body.

The Growing Pine

Benefits: Kidneys.

Start Position:

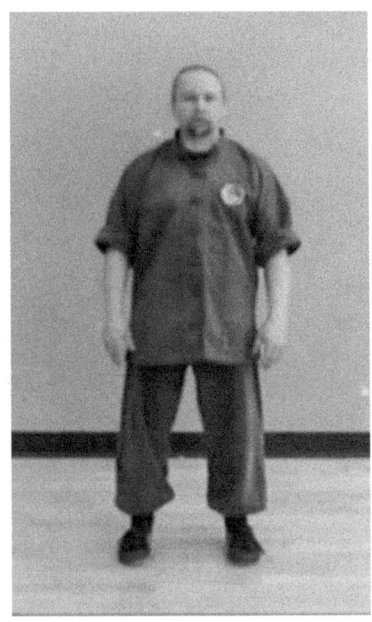

Stance: Remain in Bear stance throughout this exercise.
Posture: Arms relaxed at sides, head in neutral position.

The Growing Pine (continued)

Breathing In:

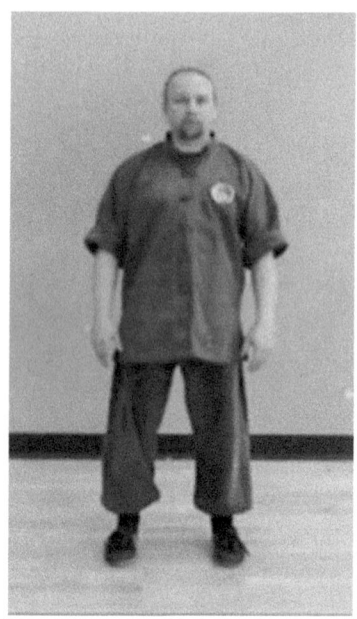

Posture: Extend upwards through the spine and at the same time extend the fingertips downwards.

The Growing Pine (continued)

Breathing Out:

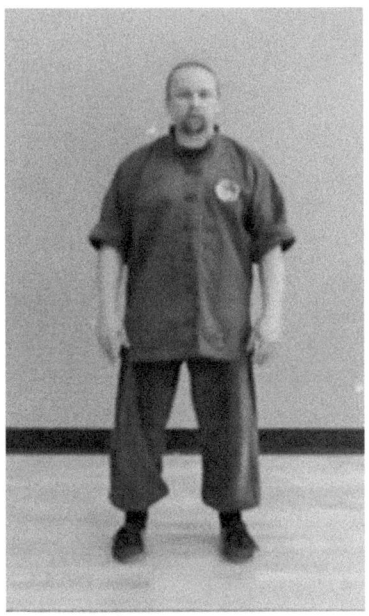

Posture: Release the extension of the spine and the arms to a neutral position.

Notes: Repeat 8 times.

Happy Day

Benefits: Heart

Start Position:

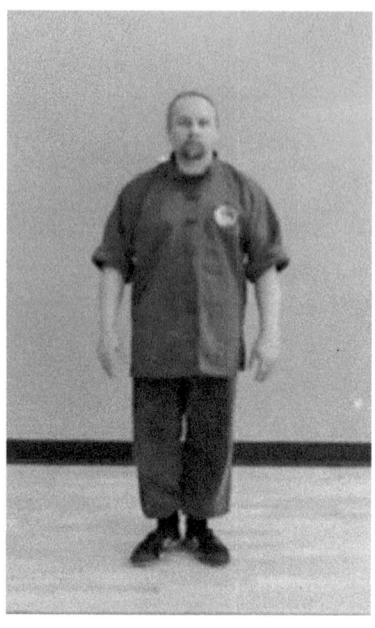

Stance: Remain in Eagle stance throughout this exercise.
Posture: Arms relaxed at sides, head in neutral position.

Happy Day (continued)

Breathing In

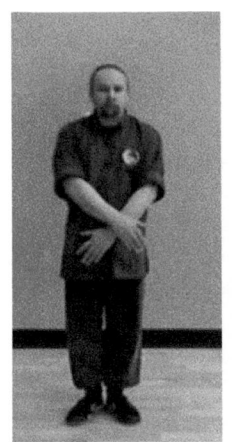 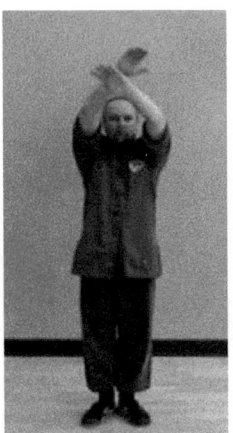 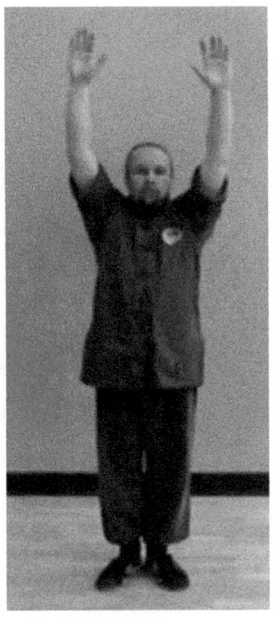

Posture: The arms come up in front of the body, initially with the palms facing inwards towards the body. As the arms come up they cross in front of the body and the palms turn to face away from the body (forwards). The arms continue upwards until they are extended above the head with the fingers pointing towards the sky.

Happy Day (continued)

Breathing Out:

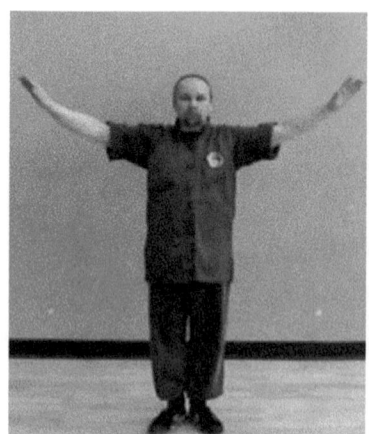
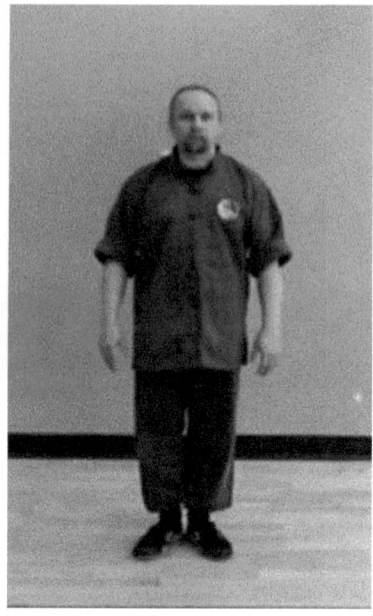

Posture: The arms continue their circles to come down and away from the body with the palms facing downwards, until they return to a neutral position by the sides.

Happy Day (continued)

Breathing In:

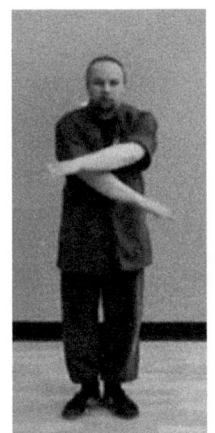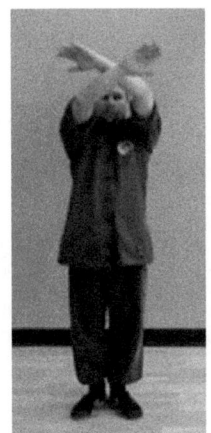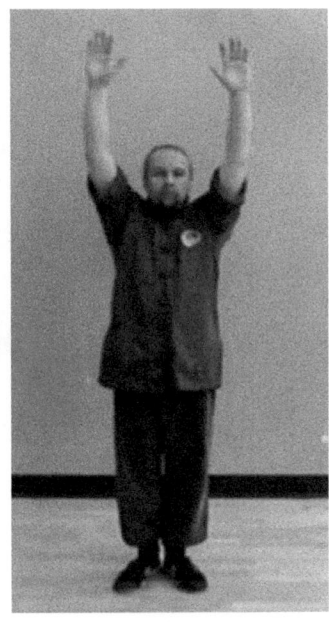

Posture: As on the first In breath the arms come up in front of the body, crossing as they rise. However, this time change the cross so that the other arm is in front. The arms continue upwards until they are extended above the head with the fingers pointing towards the sky.

Happy Day (continued)

Breathing Out:

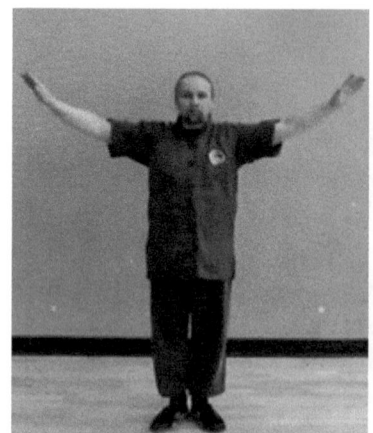
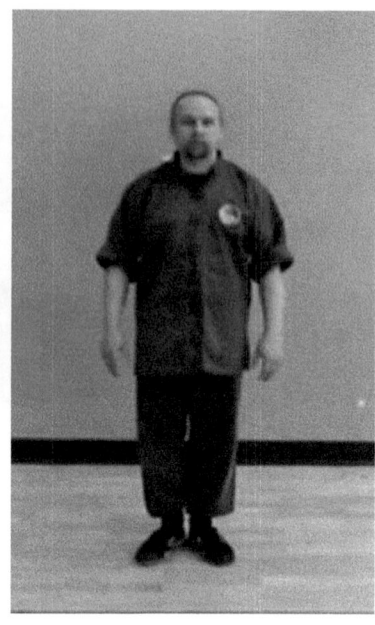

Posture: The arms continue their circles to come down and away from the body with the palms facing downwards, until they return to neutral position by the sides.

Notes: Repeat the movement 8 times, alternating the cross of the arms each time (so if the left arm is on the inside on the 1st in breath, then the right arm will be on the 2nd and so on).

Horsemanship

Benefits: Heart

Start Position:

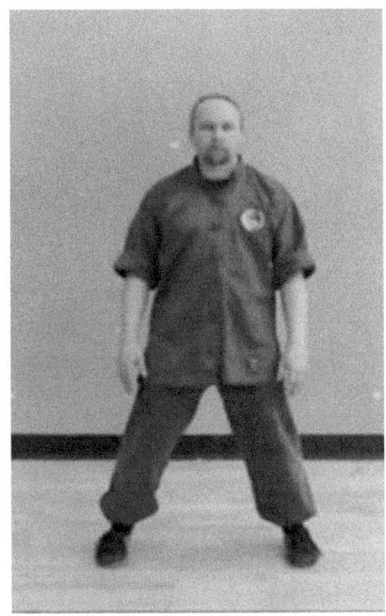

Stance: Remain in Riding Horse stance throughout the exercise.
Posture: Arms relaxed at sides, head neutral.

Horsemanship (continued)

Breathing In:

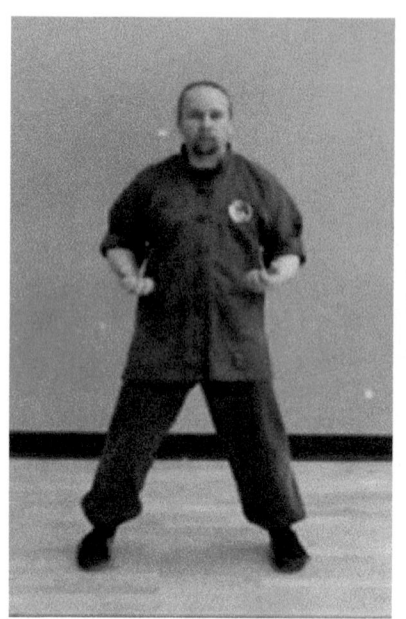 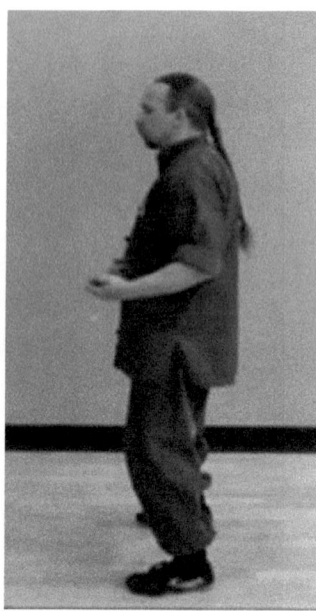

Posture: The hands come up into soft fists, palms up beside the hips.

Horsemanship (continued)

Breathing Out:

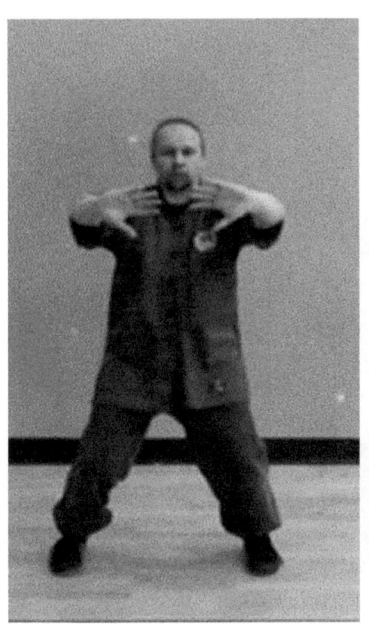 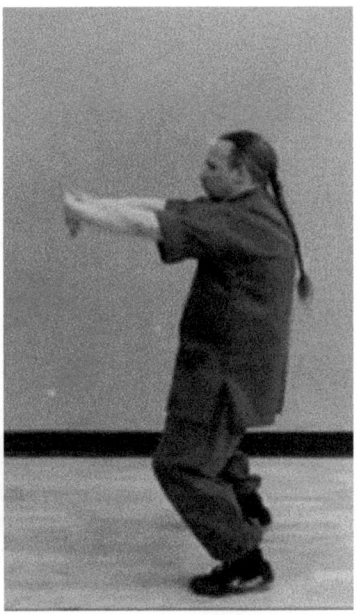

Posture: The hands 'push' out to the front to shoulder height, with the palms facing away from the body and the fingertips directed towards each other. Sink in the stance, into a deep Riding Horse as the hands push forwards.

Horsemanship (continued)

Breathing In:

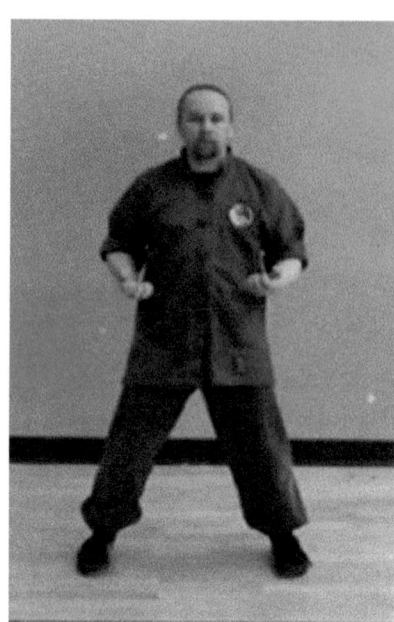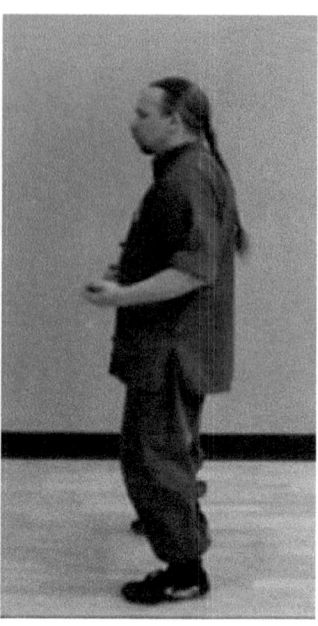

Posture: The hands return to soft fists, palms up beside the hips. Raise in the stance to come back to a 'normal' Riding Horse.

Notes: Repeat out and in breaths until you have done 8 repetitions. To finish, lower the hands to the sides to a relaxed, neutral position whilst breathing out.

Move the Rainbow

Benefits: Liver, Spleen

Start Position:

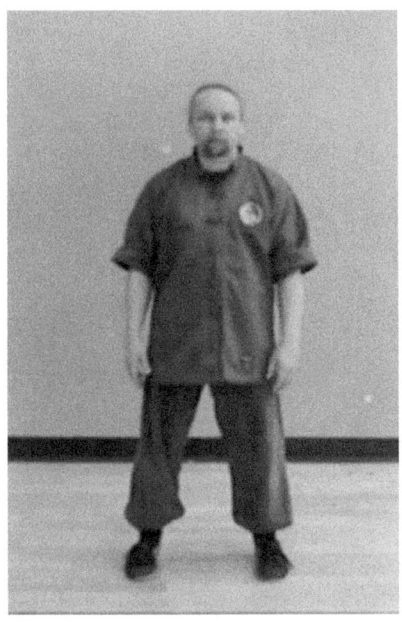

Stance: Begin in Bear stance.
Posture: Arms relaxed at sides, head neutral.

Move the Rainbow (continued)

Breathing In:

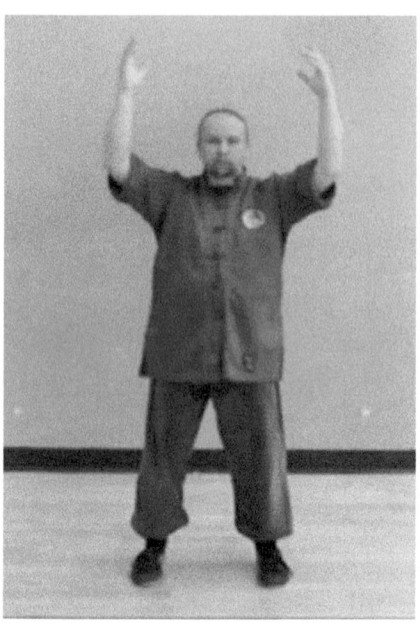

Stance: Remaining in Bear stance.
Posture: The arms lift up and out (to the sides, palms upwards) until palms face each other as if holding a 'ball' above head height.

Move the Rainbow (continued)

Breathing Out:

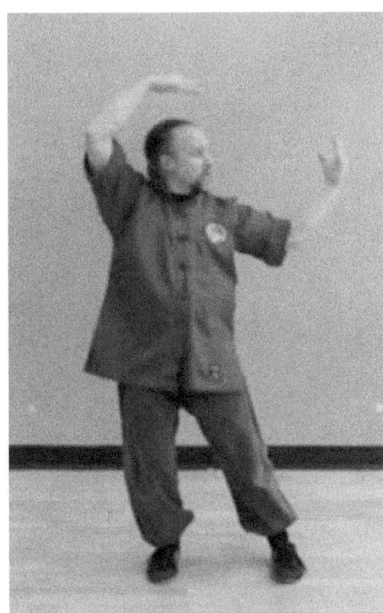

Move hips in a infinity symbol shape circular motion move arms by moving body

Stance: Shift the weight onto the right leg to come into a Leopard stance.

Posture: Lower the left arm out to the side until the hand is at head height with the palm towards the head. Turn the head to look towards the left palm. The right hand also lowers to the left so that the palm is directed towards the top of the head.

Move the Rainbow (continued)

Breathing In:

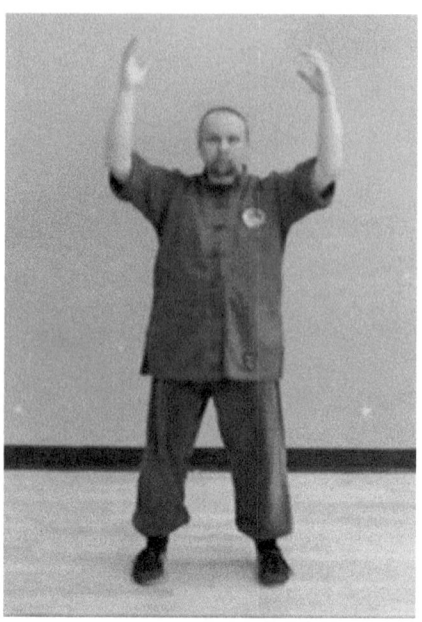

Stance: Centre the weight back onto both legs to return to Bear stance.

Posture: The hands return to holding the 'ball' above the head and the head returns to a neutral position looking forwards.

Move the Rainbow (continued)

Breathing Out:

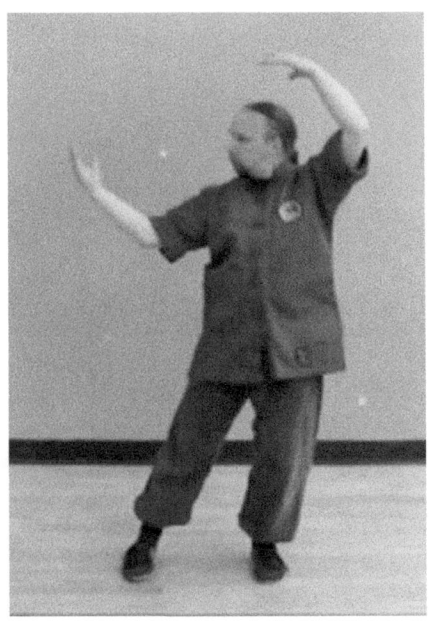

Stance: Shift the weight onto the left leg to come into a Leopard stance.

Posture: Lower the right arm out to the side until the hand is at head height with the palm towards the head. Turn the head to look towards the right palm. The left hand also lowers to the left so that the palm is directed towards the top of the head.

Move the Rainbow (continued)

Breathing In:

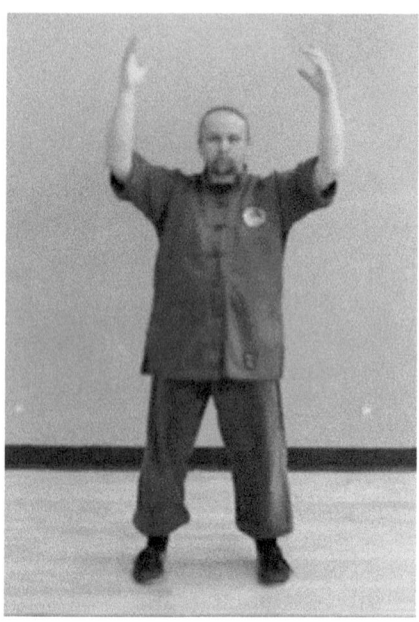

Stance: Centre the weight back onto both legs to return to Bear stance.

Posture: The hands return to holding the 'ball' above the head and the head returns to a neutral position looking forwards.

Notes: Repeat the pattern until you have moved to each side 4 or 8 times.

Move the Rainbow (continued)

Breathing Out:

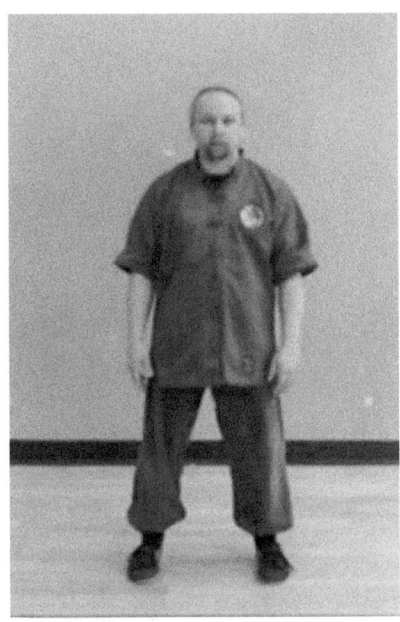

Stance: Remain in Bear stance.
Posture: Lower the arms to the sides to neutral position by the sides.

The Moving Mirror

Benefits: Kidneys, Liver, Spleen.

Start Position:

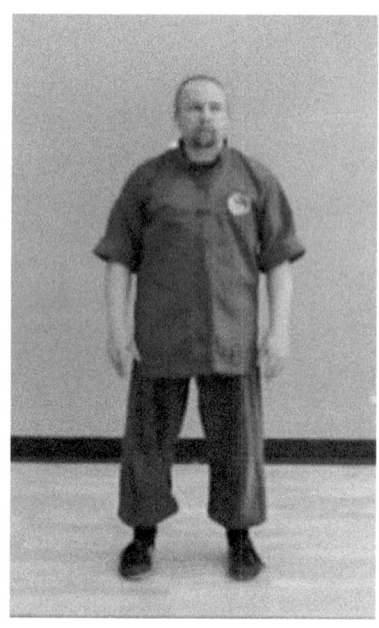

Stance: Remain in Bear stance throughout this exercise.
Posture: Arms relaxed at sides, head in neutral position.

The Moving Mirror (continued)

Breathing In:

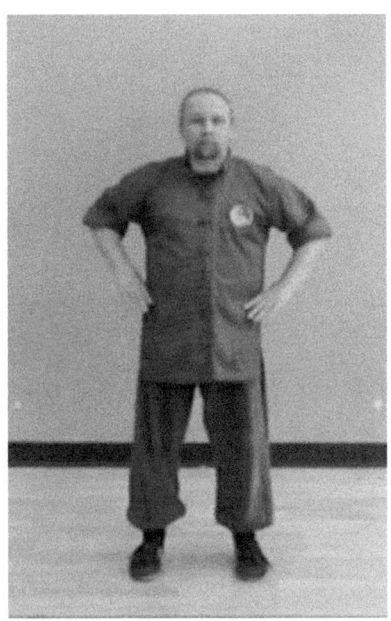

Posture: The hands come up to rest against the body above the hips – thumbs behind the body and fingers to the front with the palms downwards (making contact between the Hegu point and the body). The hands then remain in this position throughout the exercise.

The Moving Mirror (continued)

Breathing Out:

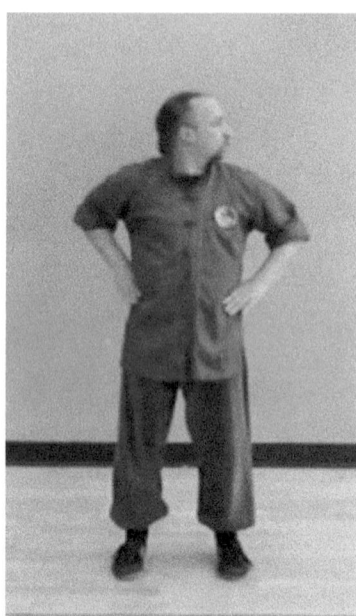

Posture: Hands remain in position. Head turns to look to left, without turning the shoulders.

The Moving Mirror (continued)

Breathing In:

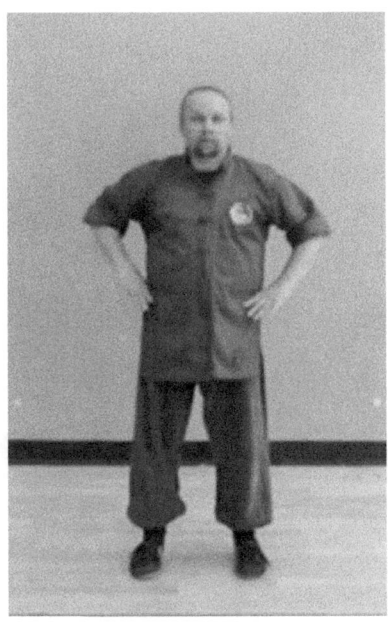

Posture: The hands remain in position. The head returns to a neutral position looking forwards.

The Moving Mirror (continued)

Breathing Out:

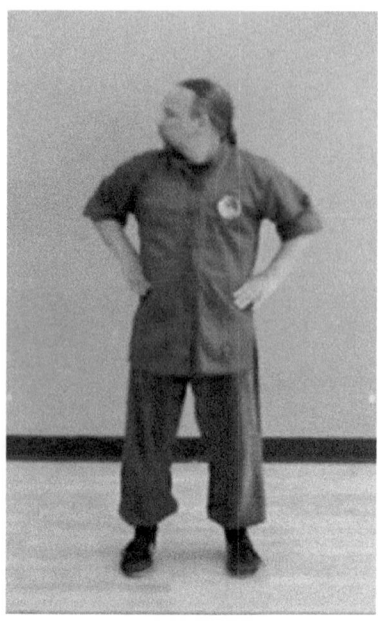

Posture: Hands remain in position. Head turns to look to right, without turning the shoulders.

The Moving Mirror (continued)

Breathing In:

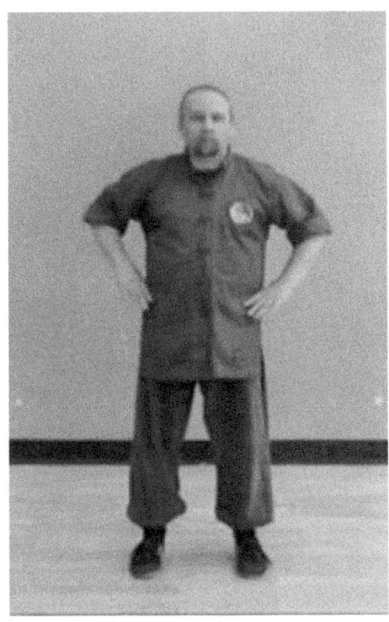

Posture: The hands remain in position. The head returns to a neutral position looking forwards.

The Moving Mirror (continued)

Breathing Out:

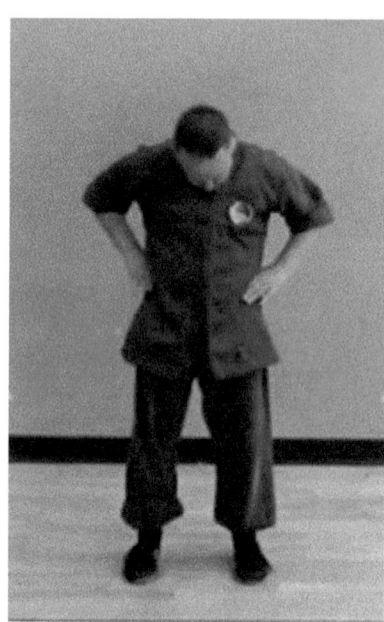 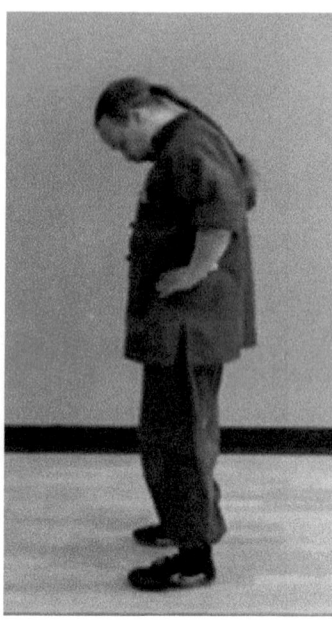

Posture: Head lowers to look downwards, extending the back of the neck without compressing the front of the neck.

The Moving Mirror (continued)

Breathing In:

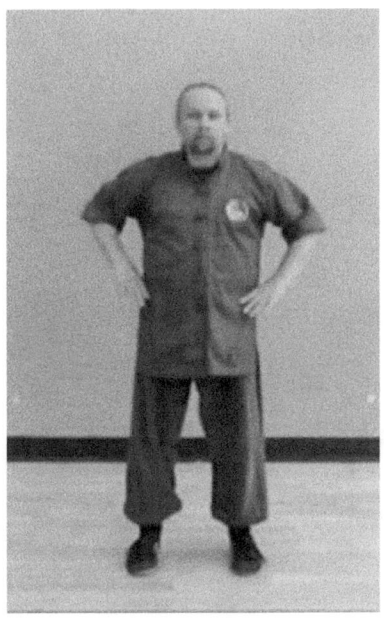

Posture: The hands remain in position. The head returns to a neutral position looking forwards.

The Moving Mirror (continued)

Breathing Out:

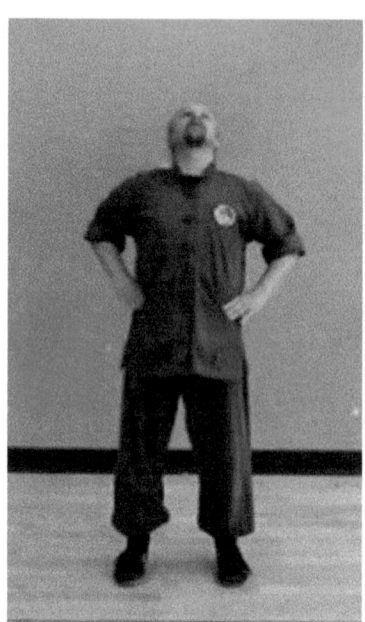 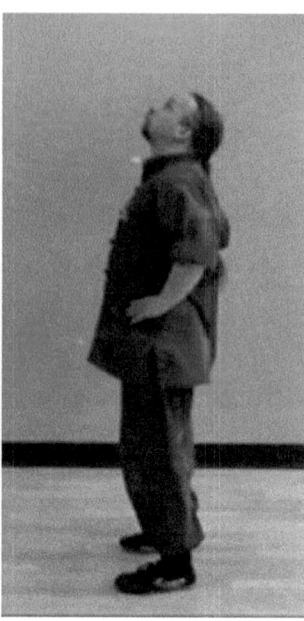

Posture: Head lifts to look upwards, extending the front of the neck and without compressing the back of the neck.

The Moving Mirror (continued)

Breathing In:

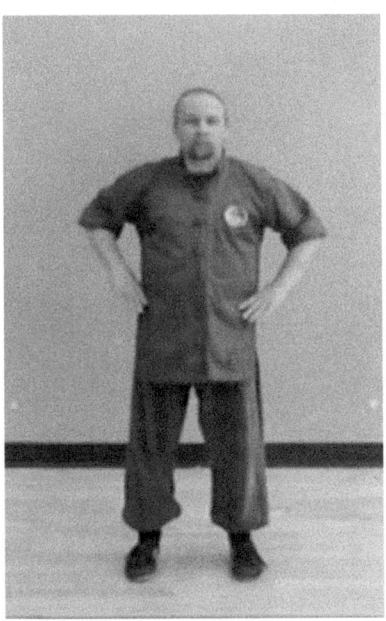

Posture: The hands remain in position. The head returns to a neutral position looking forwards.

The Moving Mirror (continued)

Breathing Out:

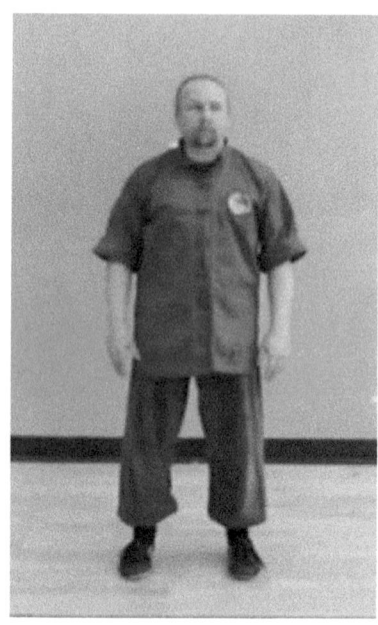

Posture: The hands lower to the sides to a neutral position.

Notes: This is an exercise where it is very important not to over-stretch – only take the movements as far as they can go comfortably without introducing tension. As the head turns to each side, be aware of the 'spiraling upwards' feeling of the twist of the spine. During the forwards and backwards 'leans', be particularly careful not to compress the opposite aspect of the neck from the stretched aspect.

Part the Waves

Benefits: Heart and Kidneys

Start Position:

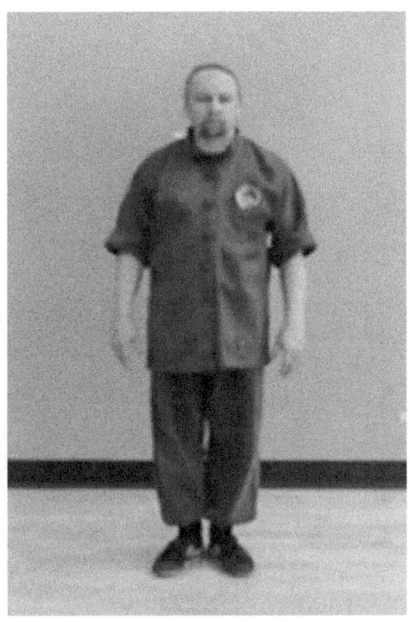

Stance: Begin in Eagle stance.
Posture: Hands relaxed at sides.

Part the Waves (continued)

Breathing In:

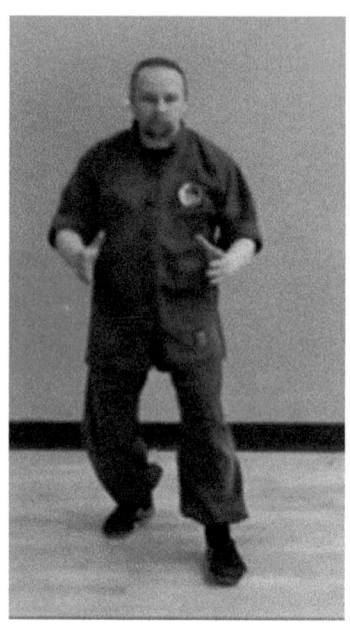 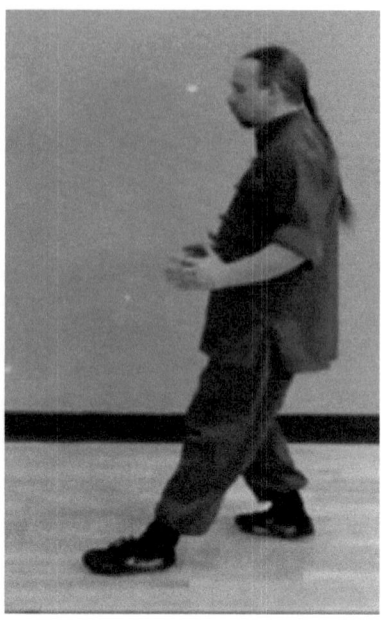

Stance: Step the left foot forwards into a Duck stance ensuring that the weight remains on the back foot.

Posture: The hands come up to palms facing each other in front of the abdomen, as if holding a ball.

Part the Waves (continued)

Breathing Out:

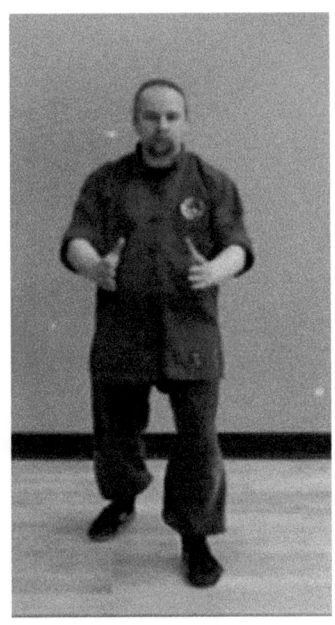 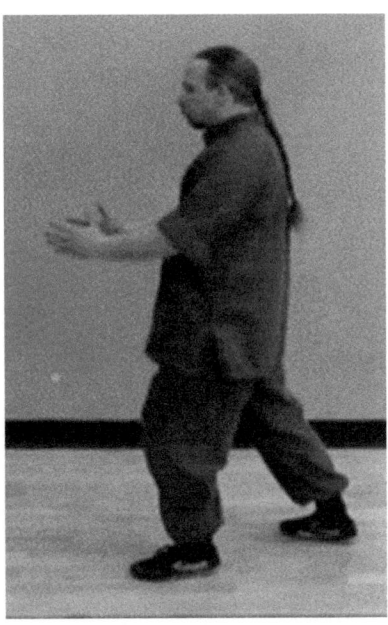

Stance: Shift the weight forwards into a Dragon stance.
Posture: The hands extend forwards with the fingertips leading, compressing the 'ball' as they extend – so moving the 'ball' away in front of the body and making it smaller.

Part the Waves (continued)

Breathing In:

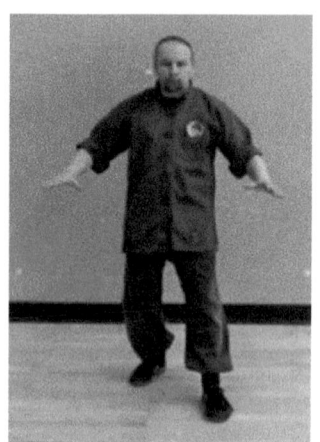
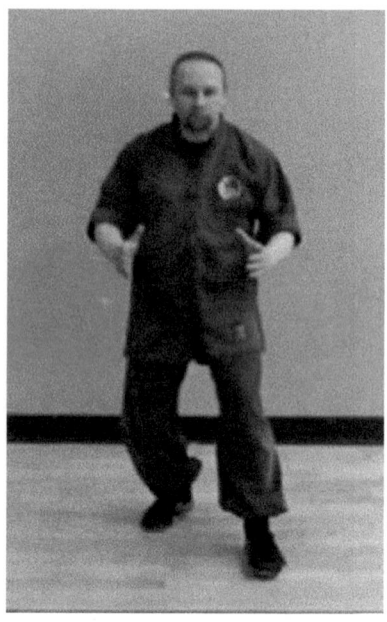

Stance: The weight shifts back into Duck stance.
Posture: The hands extend a little further forward and turn palms downwards. The hands then circle out and away from the body before continuing their circles to return to holding the 'ball' in front of the abdomen.

Notes: Repeat Out and In breaths until you have come forward into the Left Dragon stance 4 or 8 times. Then during the next In breath, follow the instructions on the next page.

Part the Waves (continued)

Breathing In:

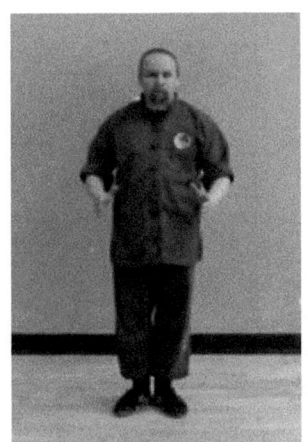 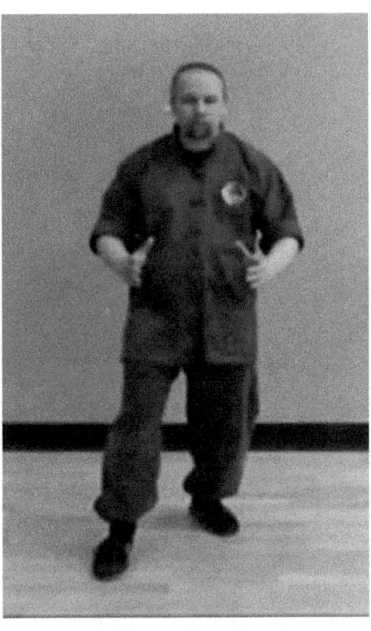

Stance: Draw the weight onto the back foot and then step the left foot back into Eagle stance. Extend the right foot forwards into a Right Duck stance, remembering to keep the weight in the back foot.

Posture: The hands extend a little further forward and turn palms downwards. The hands then circle out and away from the body before continuing their circles to return to holding the 'ball' in front of the abdomen.

Part the Waves (continued)

Breathing Out:

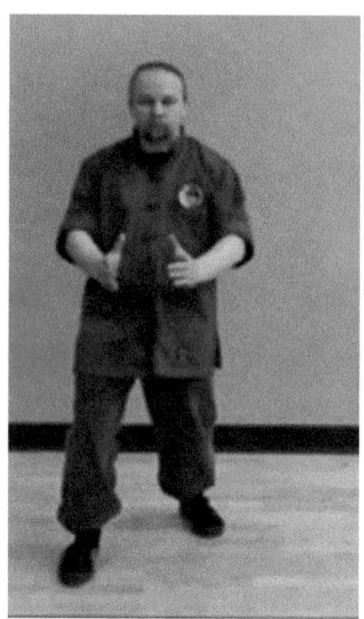 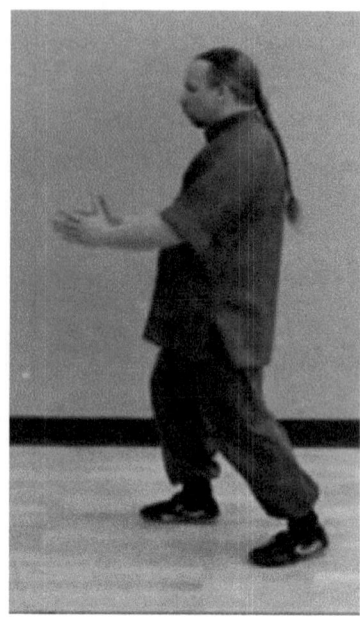

Stance: Shift the weight forwards into a Dragon stance.
Posture: The hands extend forwards with the fingertips leading, compressing the 'ball' as they extend – so moving the 'ball' away in front of the body and making it smaller.

Part the Waves (continued)

Breathing In:

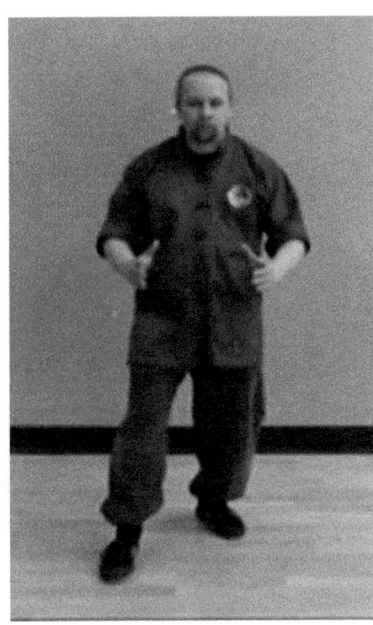 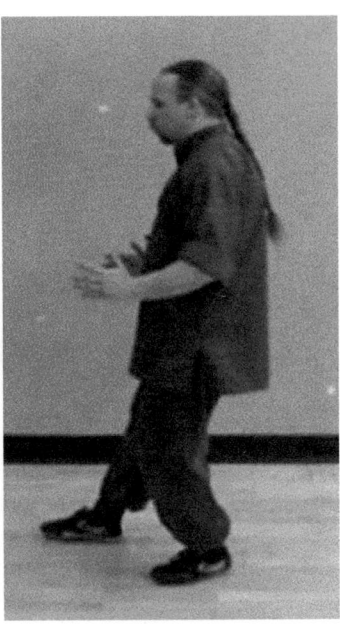

Stance: The weight shifts back into Duck stance.
Posture: The hands extend a little further forward and turn palms downwards. The hands then circle out and away from the body before continuing their circles to return to holding the 'ball' in front of the abdomen.

Notes: Again, repeat on the right side until you have done the same number of repetitions that you did on the left side. On the final In breath, draw the foot back to come back into Eagle stance.

Part the Waves (continued)

Breathing Out:

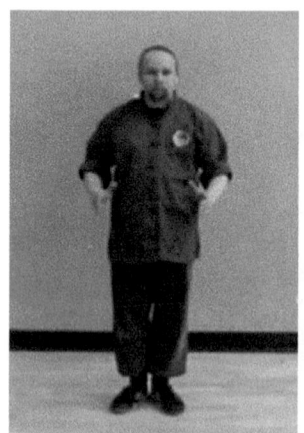 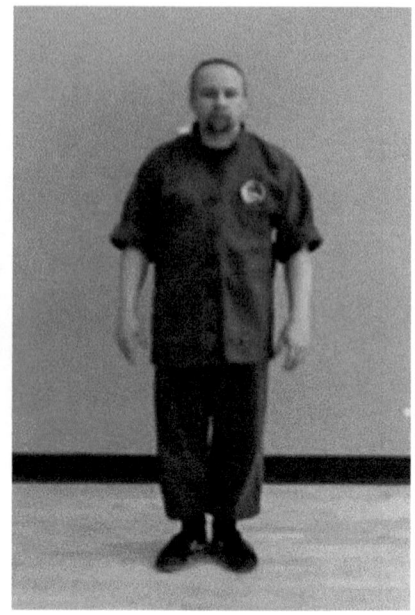

Stance: Remain in Eagle stance.
Posture: The arms lower to a neutral position by the sides.

Notes: As the arms return to holding a ball in front of the abdomen, they circle back at waist height – it can be useful to imagine standing waist deep in water and the hands glide back along the surface of the water.

Play the Shuttlecock

Benefits: Liver, Spleen, Kidneys

Start Position:

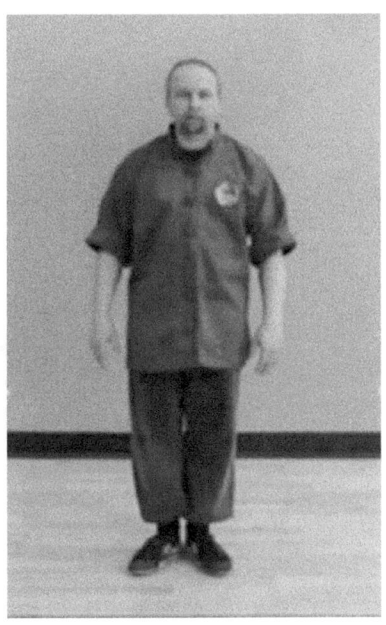

Stance: Begin in Eagle stance.
Posture: Hands relaxed at sides.

Play the Shuttlecock (continued)

Breathing In:

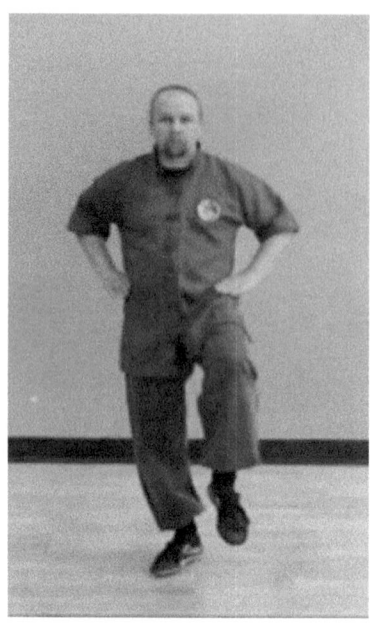

Stance: Lift the left leg into Crane stance.
Posture: The hands come up to rest against the body above the hips – thumbs behind the body and fingers to the front with the palms downwards. The hands then remain in this position throughout the exercise.

Play the Shuttlecock (continued)

Breathing Out:

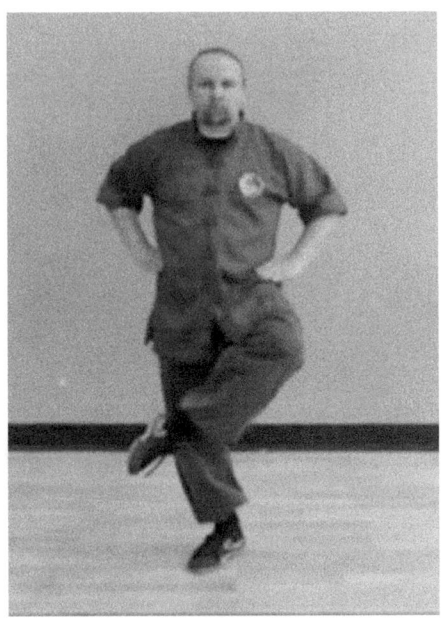

Stance: Maintaining the position of the knee, bring the lower left leg 'inwards' to the right turning the sole of the foot towards the ceiling as much as possible.
Posture: Hands remain in position on waist.

Play the Shuttlecock (continued)

Breathing In:

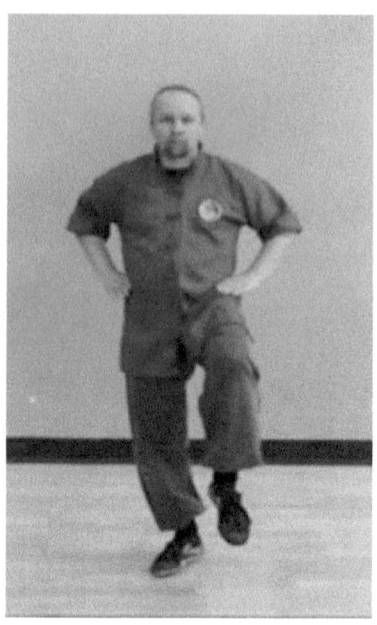

Stance: Bring the lower left leg back into a normal Crane stance position.
Posture: Hands remain in position on waist.

Play the Shuttlecock (continued)

Breathing Out:

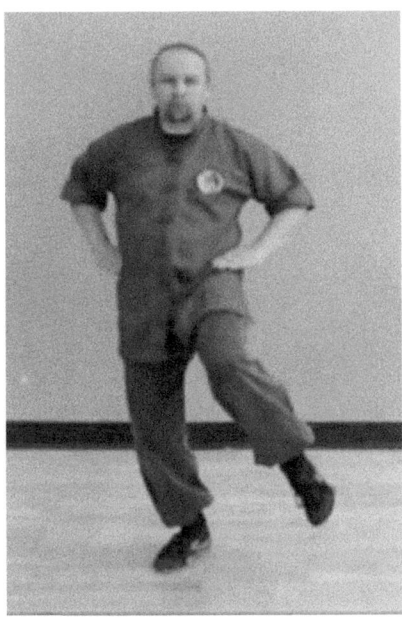

Stance: Maintaining the position of the knee, bring the lower left leg 'outwards' to the left aiming to turn the sole of the foot towards the ceiling as much as possible.
Posture: Hands remain in position on waist.

Play the Shuttlecock (continued)

Breathing In:

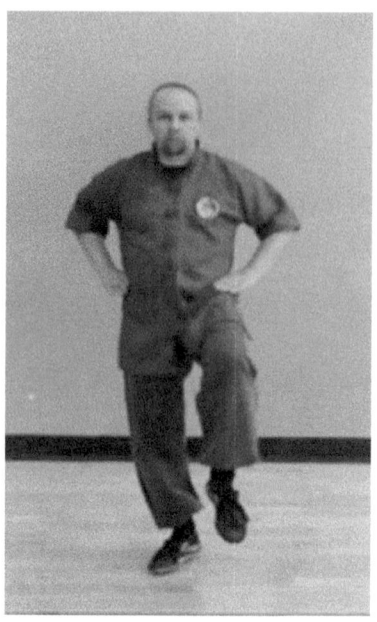

Stance: Bring the lower left leg back into a normal Crane stance position.
Posture: Hands remain in position on waist.

Play the Shuttlecock (continued)

Breathing Out:

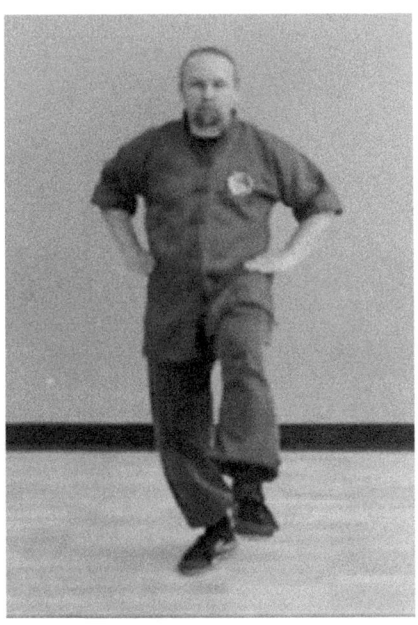

Stance: Extend the lower left leg forwards into Dog stance (leg extended to the front, maintaining slight bend in the knee and no higher than thigh parallel to floor). Dropping the toes at the end of the movement to 'step' heel-toe.
Posture: Hands remain in position on waist.

Play the Shuttlecock (continued)

Breathing In:

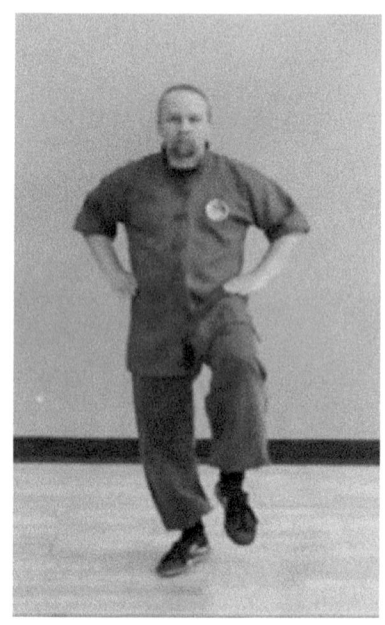

Stance: Bring the left leg back into a Crane stance position.
Posture: Hands remain in position on waist.

Play the Shuttlecock (continued)

Breathing Out:

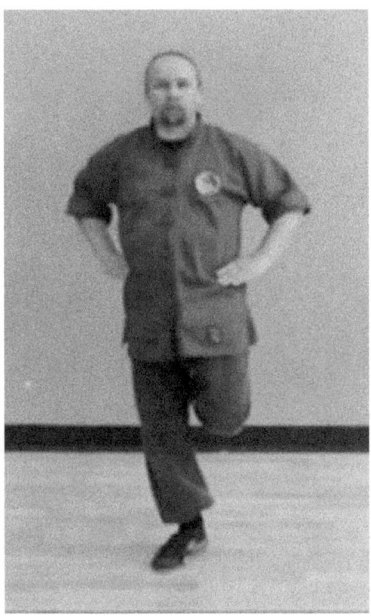

Stance: Bring the left foot up behind the body with the heel towards the buttock, extending the toes upwards.
Posture: Hands remain in position on waist.

Play the Shuttlecock (continued)

Breathing In:

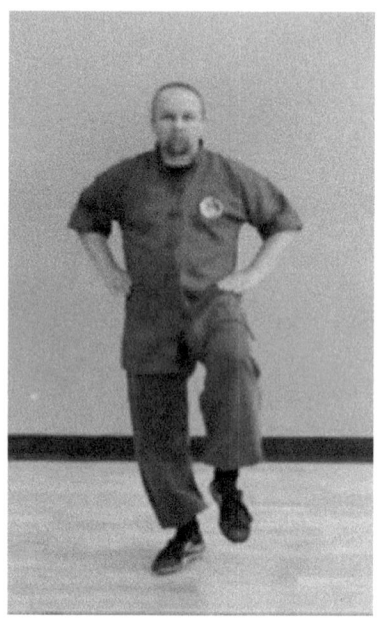

Stance: Bring the left leg back into a normal Crane stance.
Posture: Hands remain in position on waist.

Play the Shuttlecock (continued)

Breathing Out:

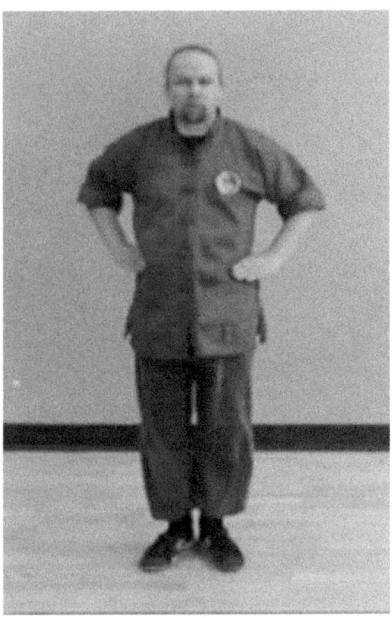

Stance: Lower the left leg back down into Eagle stance.
Posture: Hands remain in position on waist.

Play the Shuttlecock (continued)

Breathing In:

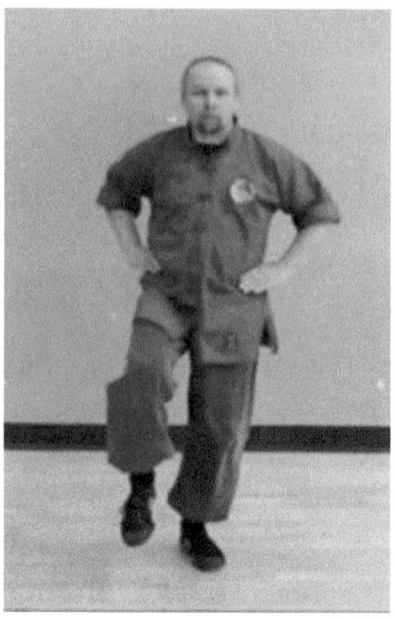

Stance: Bring the right leg up into a Crane stance.
Posture: Hands remain in position on waist.

Notes: Repeat each of the steps as outlined above but with the right leg this time. Then, if desired, repeat the exercise on each leg until 4 or 8 repetitions are completed. After your last repetition the final 'Out' breath should complete the exercise as follows:

Play the Shuttlecock (continued)

Breathing Out:

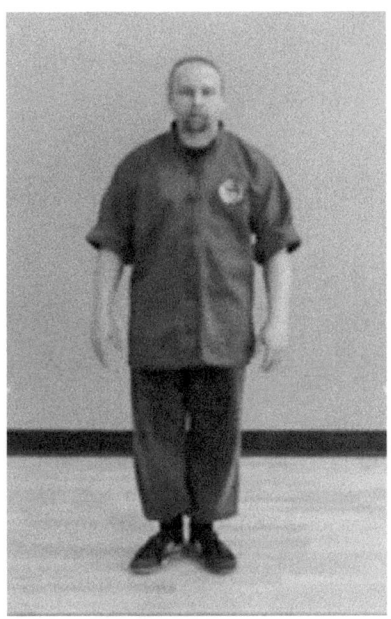

Stance: Lower the leg back down into Eagle stance.
Posture: Hands lower back down into a neutral position by the sides.

Push the Wave

Benefits: Heart and Kidneys.

Start Position:

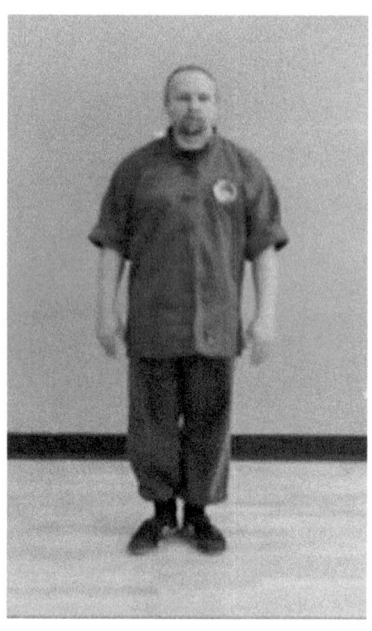

Stance: Begin in Eagle stance.
Posture: Hands relaxed at sides.

Push the Wave (continued)

Breathing In:

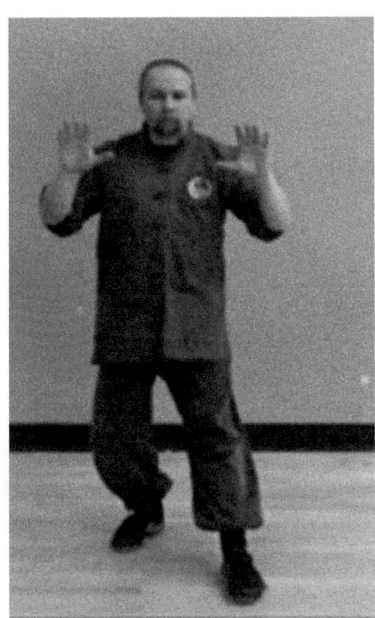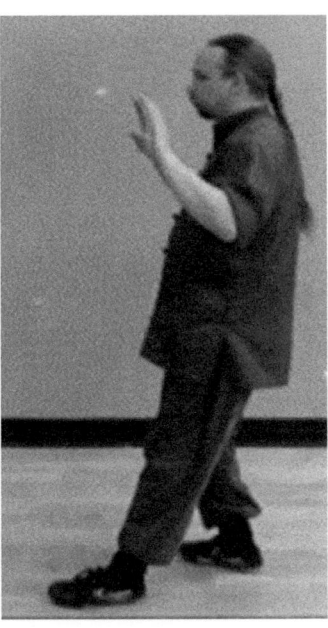

Stance: Step the left foot forwards into a Duck stance ensuring that the weight remains on the back foot.

Posture: The hands come up to palms facing away from the body in front of the shoulders (fingers pointing upwards).

Push the Wave (continued)

Breathing Out:

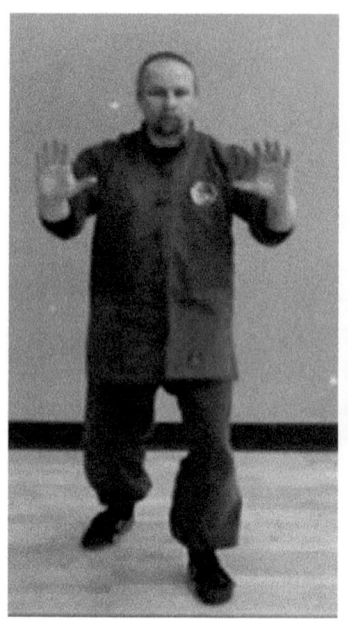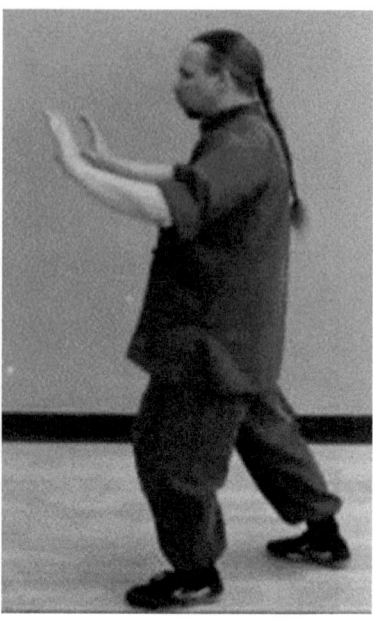

Stance: Shift the weight forwards into a Dragon stance.
Posture: The hands extend forwards 'pushing' with the palms.

Push the Wave (continued)

Breathing In:

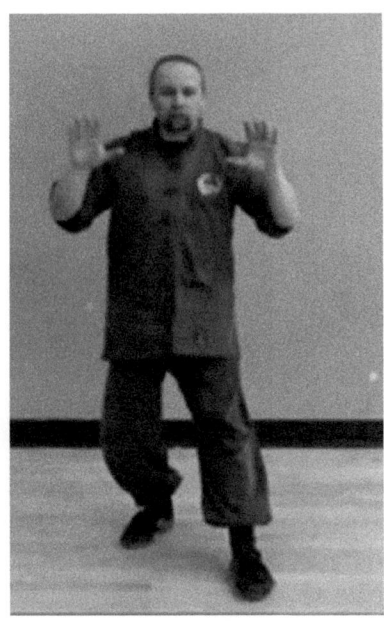 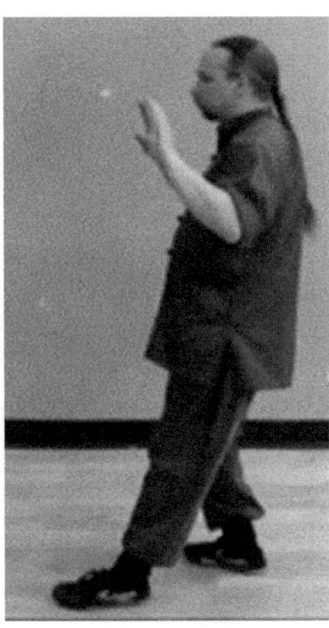

Stance: The weight shifts back into Duck stance.
Posture: Hands draw back to in front of the shoulders, palms forwards, fingertips upwards.

Notes: Repeat Out and In breaths until you have come forward into the Left Dragon stance 4 or 8 times.

Push the Wave (continued)

Breathing In:

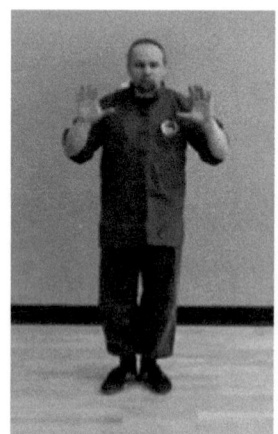
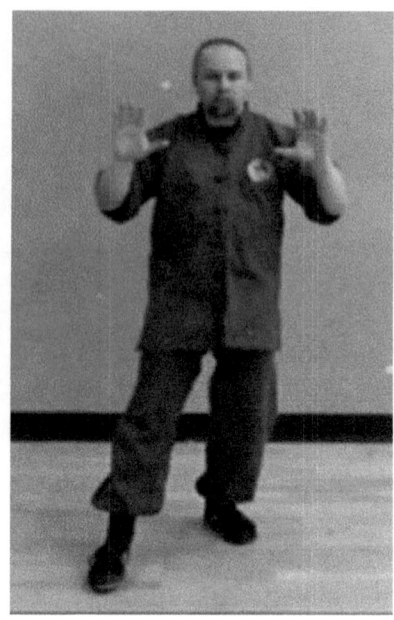

Stance: Draw the weight back into a Left Duck stance and then step the left foot back to Eagle stance. The right foot then steps forwards into Right Duck stance.
Posture: Hands draw back to in front of the shoulders, palms forwards, fingertips upwards.

Push the Wave (continued)

Breathing Out:

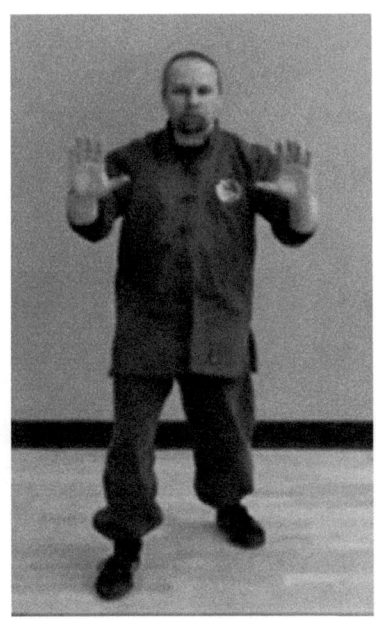 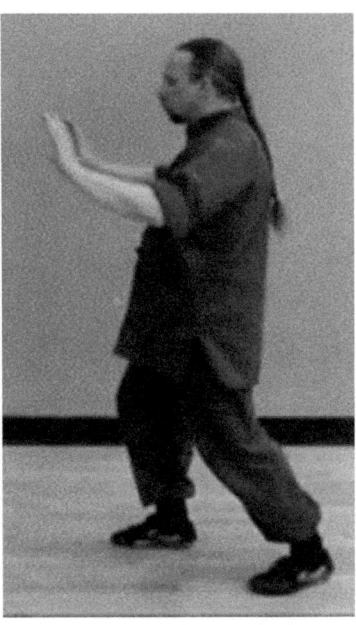

Stance: Shift the weight forwards into a Dragon stance.
Posture: The hands extend forwards 'pushing' with the palms.

Push the Wave (continued)

Breathing In:

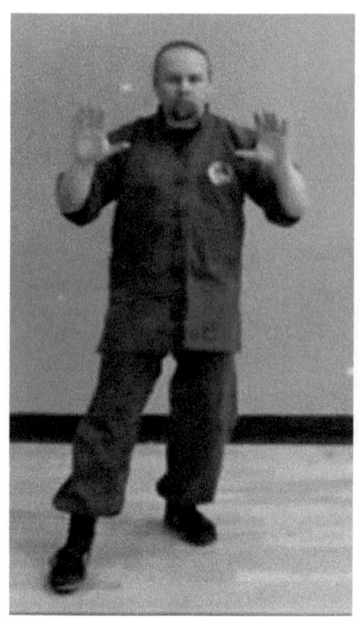 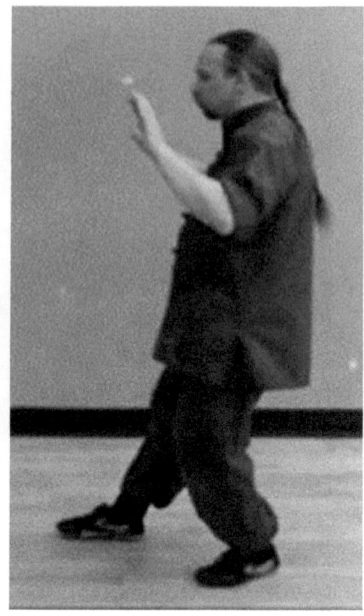

Stance: The weight shifts back into Duck stance.
Posture: Hands draw back to in front of the shoulders, palms forwards, fingertips upwards.

Notes: Again, repeat on the right side until you have done the same number of repetitions that you did on the left side.

Push the Wave (continued)

Breathing In:

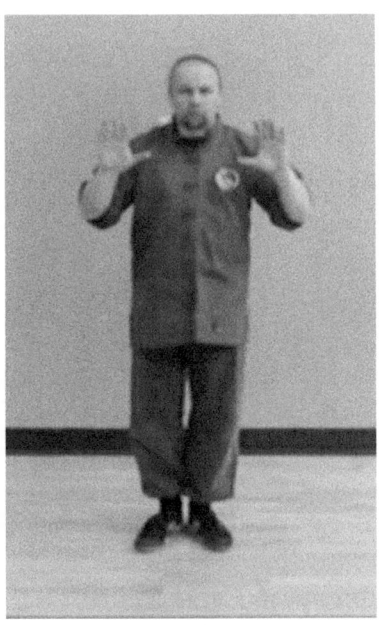

Stance: The weight shifts back into Duck stance and then draw the right foot back into Eagle stance.
Posture: Hands draw back to in front of the shoulders, palms forwards, fingertips upwards.

Push the Wave (continued)

Breathing Out:

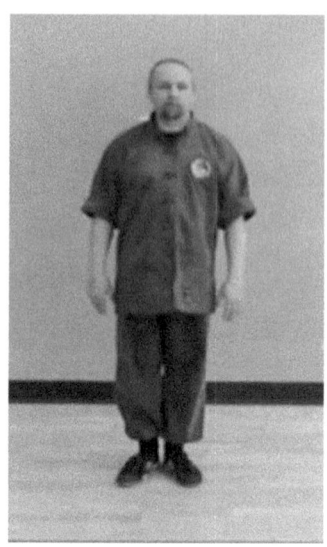

Stance: Remain in Eagle stance.
Posture: The arms lower to a neutral position by the sides.

Notes: As the arms move forwards they follow a curving path slightly down and then up, they then continue this pattern on the way back towards the body (slightly upwards and then down into position). This will give a feeling of pressing forwards 'fingers then palms.' However, do not over-exaggerate the circular motion – the hands should only go slightly below or above shoulder height during the movement.

Rock the Ball

Benefits: Kidneys

Start Position:

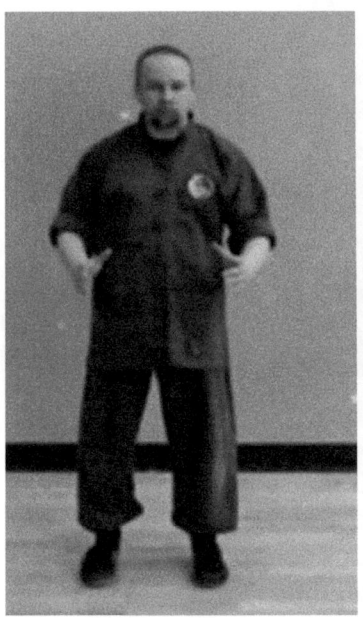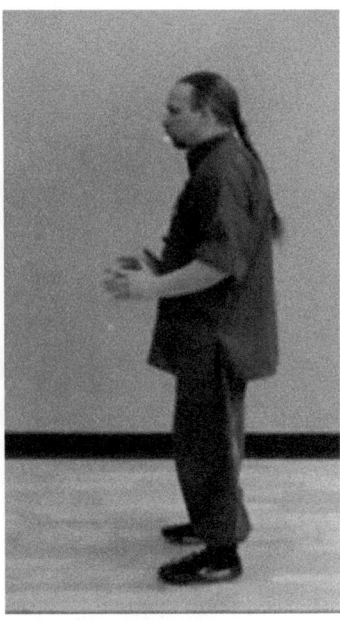

Stance: Remain in Bear stance throughout this exercise.
Posture: Hands start with the palms facing each other as if holding a 'ball' in front of the abdomen. The hands should be at Tantien height (so just below navel height).

Rock the Ball (continued)

Breathing In:

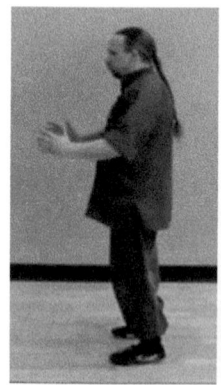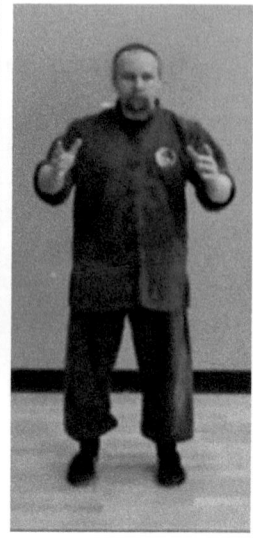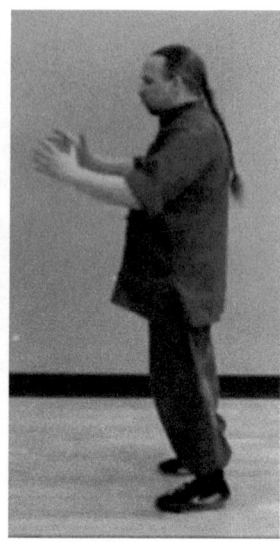

Stance: Remain in Bear stance, but rock the weight forwards slightly over the balls of the feet (not so far that the heels lift off the floor).

Posture: The hands continue to face palms towards each other as if holding a 'ball'. Raise the 'ball' to chest height, extending it slightly forward away from the body.

Rock the Ball (continued)

Breathing Out:

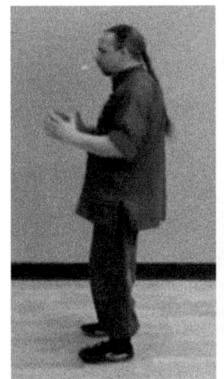
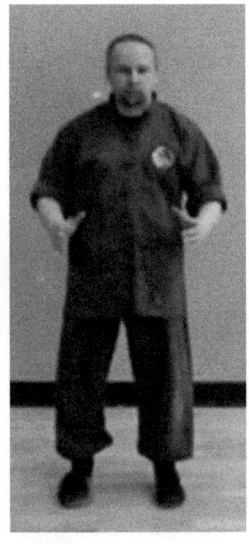
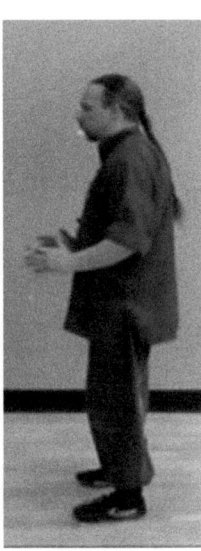

Stance: Rock the weight back across the balls of the feet to bring most of the weight onto the heels (do not lift the toes off the floor).

Posture: Hands continue to hold the 'ball'. At the top of the movement (chest height) the ball draws back in towards the body and then lowers down to in front of the abdomen as at the start of the exercise.

Notes: Repeat the exercise until you have done 8 repetitions. Be aware of the 'circular' motion that the hands follow as they move up and away and then down and in.

Rotate the Wheel

Benefits: Liver, Spleen, Kidneys.

Start Position:

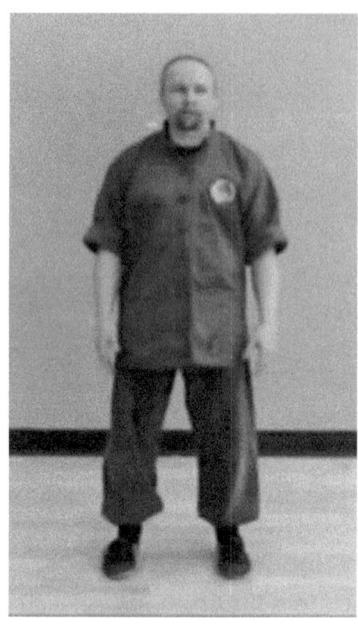

Stance: Remain in Bear stance throughout this exercise.
Posture: Arms start in a relaxed, neutral position by the sides.

Rotate the Wheel (continued)

Breathing In:

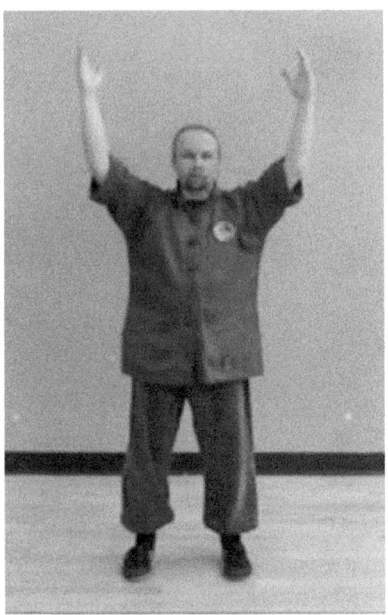

Posture: The arms come up and out to the sides before continuing upwards to finish palms facing each other as if holding a 'ball' directly above the head.

Rotate the Wheel (continued)

Breathing Out:

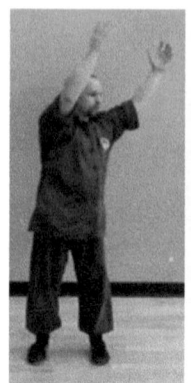
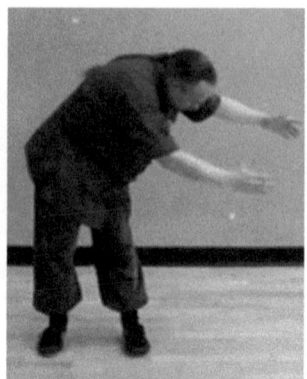
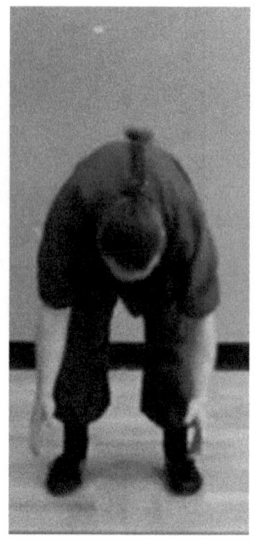

Posture: Maintaining the feeling of holding a 'ball' (so palms continue to face each other throughout), bring the arms down to the left side of the body (turning the waist to the left). Continue the movement until the fingers are pointing downwards with the 'ball' held in front of the legs and the body is leaning forward from the waist.

Rotate the Wheel (continued)

Breathing In:

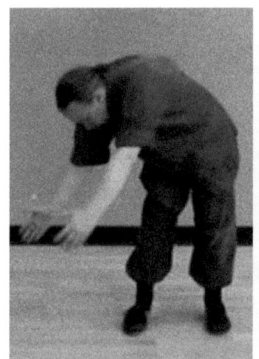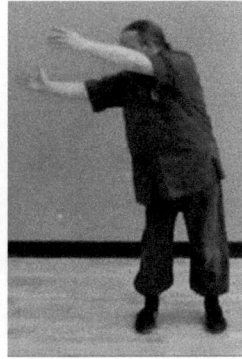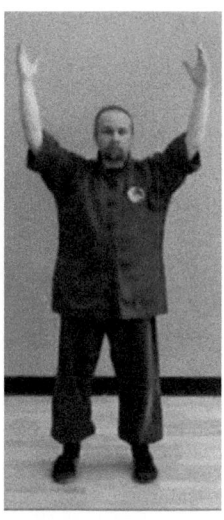

Posture: Continue the circle to bring the ball upwards, to the right-hand side of the body until the ball is once again above the head.

Notes: Repeat until you have done 4 or 8 repetitions of circling the 'ball' down and to the left and up and to the right.

Rotate the Wheel (continued)

Breathing Out:

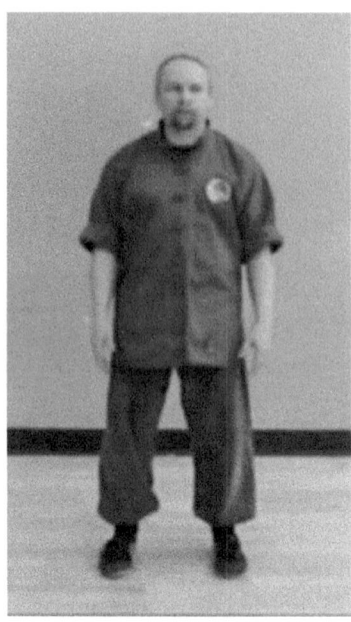

Posture: Lower the arms to the sides to a neutral, relaxed position.

Notes: Then repeat the exercise with the circle going in the opposite direction (down and right and then up and left).

Separate the Clouds

Benefits: Heart

Start Position:

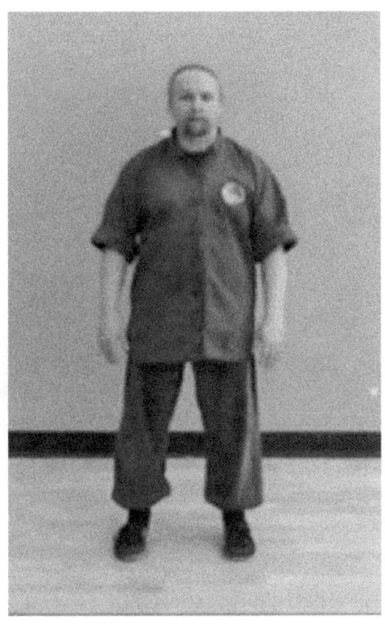

Stance: Remain in Bear stance throughout this exercise.
Posture: Arms start in a relaxed, neutral position by the sides.

Separate the Clouds (continued)

Breathing In:

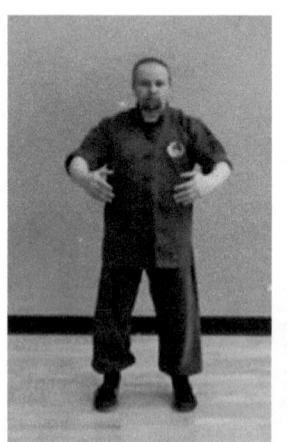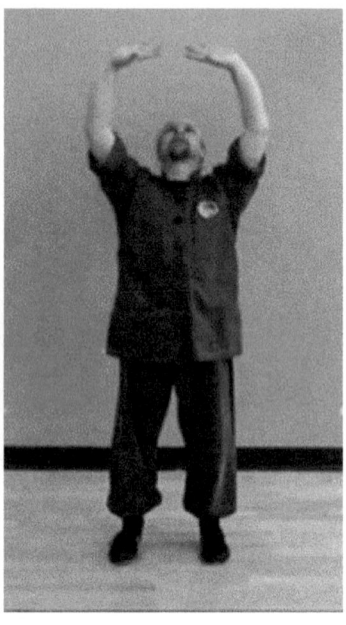

Posture: Hands come upwards to face palms inwards towards the abdomen with the fingertips pointing towards each other. Continue the upwards movement and as the hands come in front of the face, they turn to face palms away (fingertips still directed towards each other). The head now follows the hand movement, so watch the hands as the upward movement continues until the hands are above the head with the palms facing upwards.

Separate the Clouds (continued)

Breathing Out:

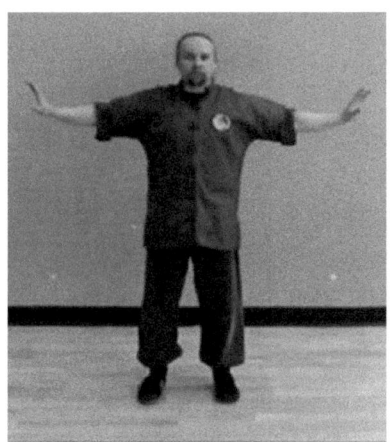
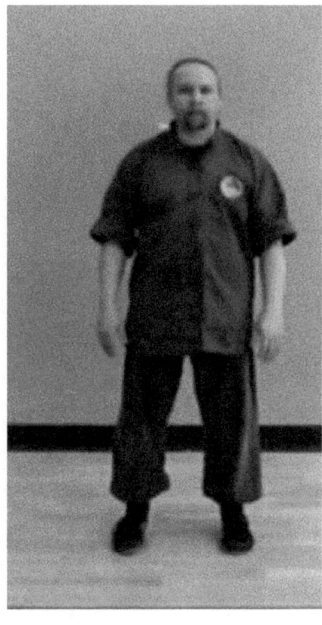

Posture: The hands separate away from each other and lower down to the sides with the palms facing downwards until the arms are in a relaxed, neutral position by sides. As the hands lower, the head also returns to a neutral position.

Notes: Repeat the exercise until you have done 8 repetitions.

Shao Gong (Large)

Benefits: Balancing Qigong

Start Position:

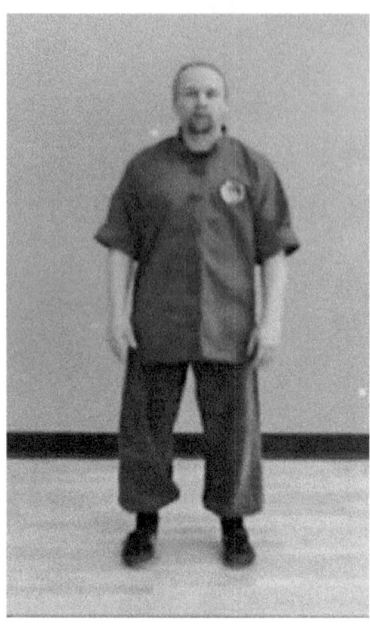

Stance: Remain in Bear stance throughout this exercise.
Posture: Arms start in a relaxed, neutral position by the sides.

Shao Gong (Large) (continued)

Breathing In:

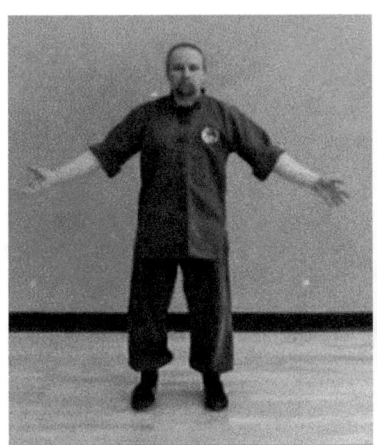
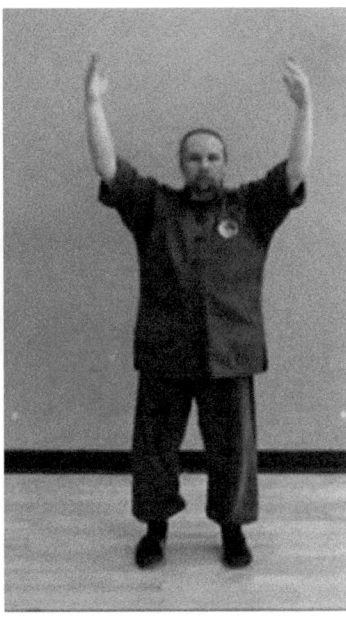

Posture: The arms come up and out to the sides (palms upwards) and then turn to palms facing towards each other above the head.

Shao Gong (Large) (continued)

Breathing Out:

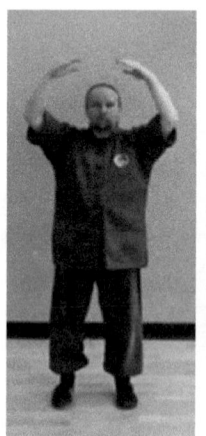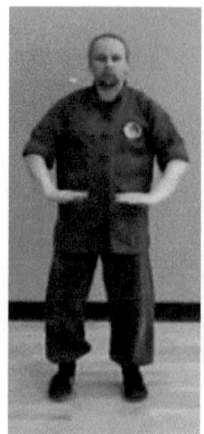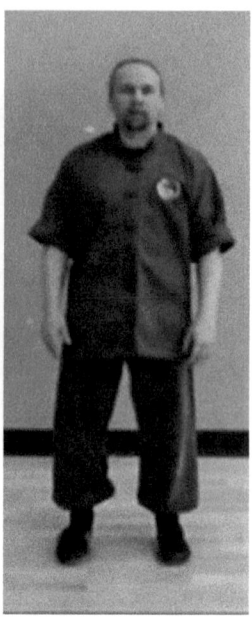

Posture: The hands 'press' downwards in front of the body (fingertips towards each other) and then lower to a neutral position by the sides.

Notes: Repeat the exercise until you have done 8 repetitions. As the arms come downwards on the out breath, think about lowering the shoulders, then the elbows and then the hands. Repeat the exercise until you have done 8 repetitions.

Shao Gong (Small)

Benefits: Balancing Qigong

Start Position:

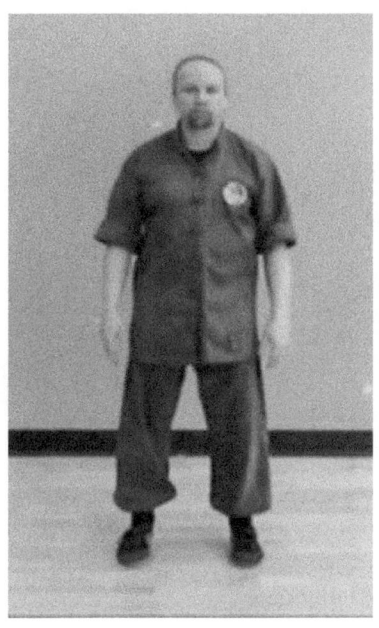

Stance: Remain in Bear stance throughout this exercise.
Posture: Arms start in a relaxed, neutral position by the sides.

Shao Gong (Small) (continued)

Breathing In:

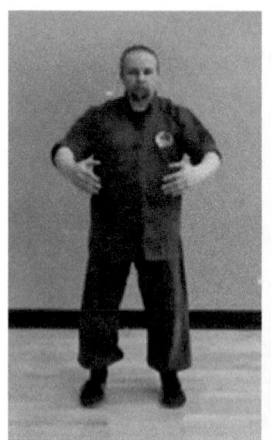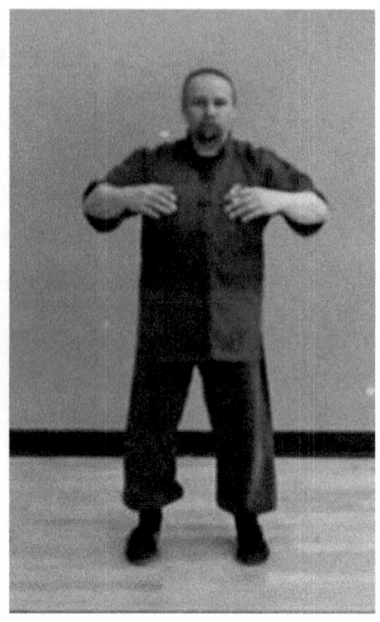

Posture: The hands circle up to a position in front of the chest with the palms down and fingertips towards each other.

Shao Gong (Small) (continued)

Breathing Out:

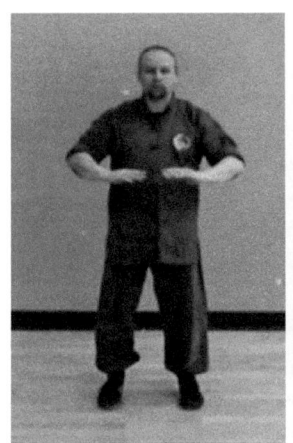
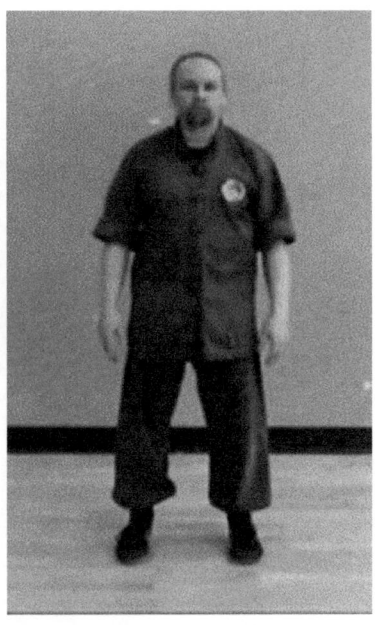

Posture: The hands press down in front of the body (fingertips towards each other, palms down) and then lower to a relaxed position by the sides.

Notes: Repeat the exercise until you have done 8 repetitions.

Step Forwards and Look Back

Benefits: Kidneys, Liver, Spleen

Start Position:

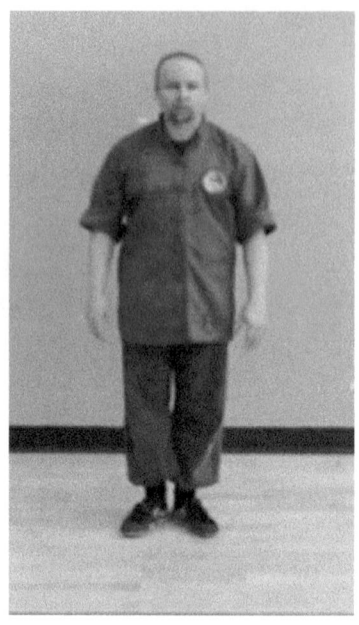

Stance: Begin in Eagle stance.
Posture: Hands relaxed at sides.

Step Forwards and Look Back (continued)

Breathing In:

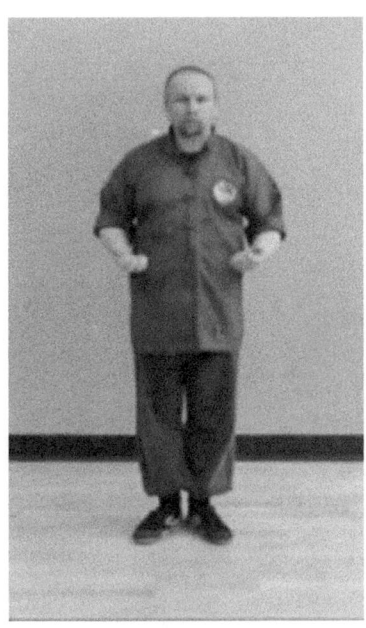

Stance: Remain in Eagle stance.
Posture: Hands come up into soft fists, palms up beside hips.

Step Forwards and Look Back (continued)

Breathing Out:

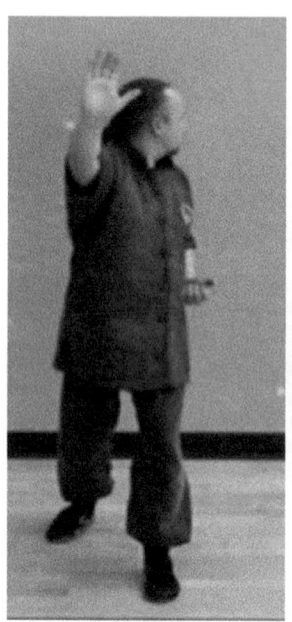 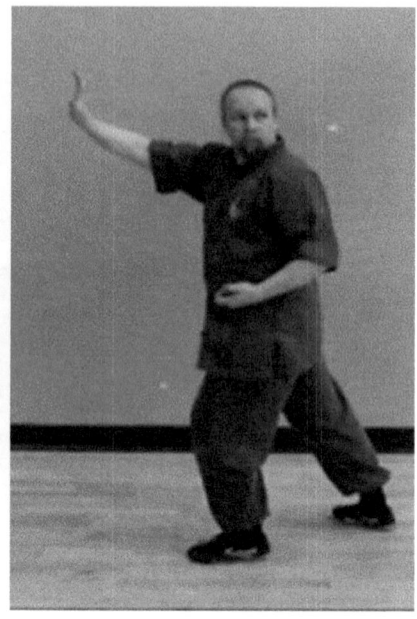

Stance: Step the left foot forwards into a Dragon stance.
Posture: The right hand opens and then extends forwards to a little above shoulder height with the palm facing forwards away from the body. The left hand stays in a fist beside the hip and the head turns to look back over the left shoulder.

Step Forwards and Look Back (continued)

Breathing In:

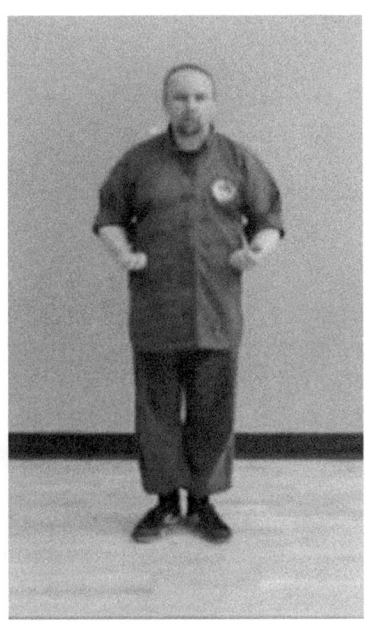

Stance: Draw the left foot back in to Eagle stance.
Posture: The right hand returns to a soft fist, palm up beside the hip. The head returns to neutral.

Step Forwards and Look Back (continued)

Breathing Out:

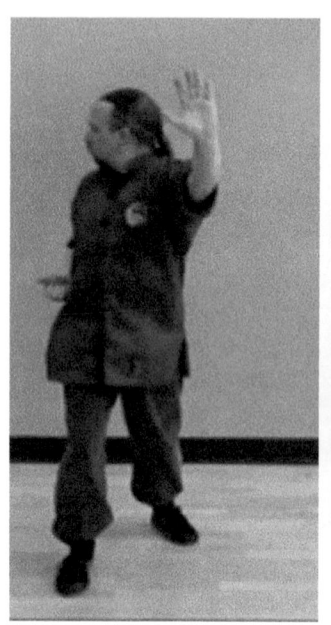 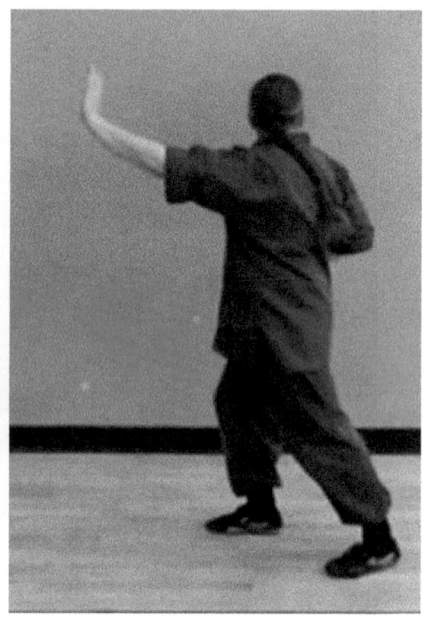

Stance: Step the right foot forwards into a Dragon stance.

Posture: The left hand opens and then extends forwards to a little above shoulder height with the palm facing forwards away from the body. The right hand stays in a fist beside the hip and the head turns to look back over the right shoulder.

Step Forwards and Look Back (continued)

Breathing In:

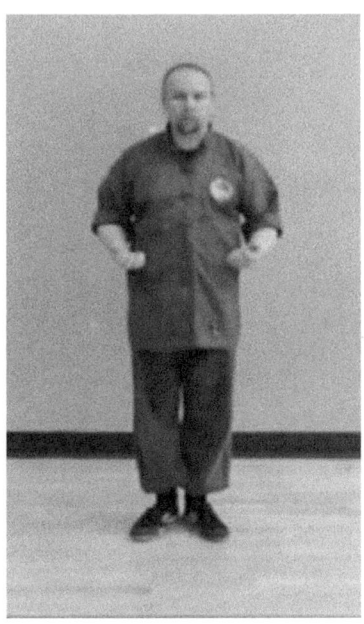

Stance: Draw the right foot back in to Eagle stance.
Posture: The left hand returns to a soft fist, palm up beside the hip. The head returns to neutral.

Notes: Repeat until you have come forward into each Dragon stance 4 or 8 times.

Step Forwards and Look Back (continued)

Breathing Out:

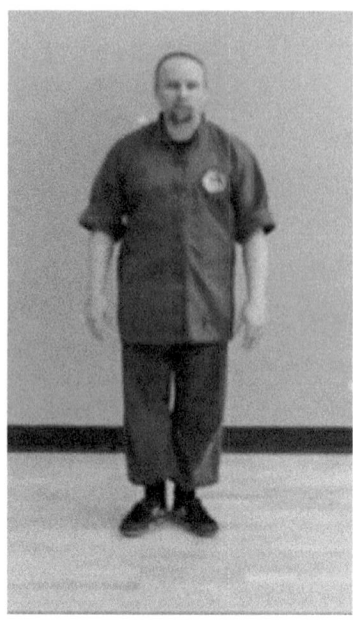

Stance: Remain in Eagle stance.
Posture: The hands open and lower to neutral position by the sides.

Notes: Be aware of the spiraling motion of the hand as it extends forwards and as it returns to beside the hip.

Stop the Five Seasons

Benefits: Balancing Qigong

Start Position:

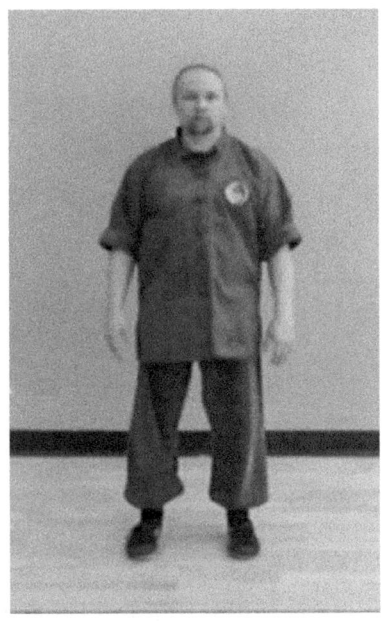

Stance: Remain in Bear stance throughout this exercise.
Posture: Arms start in a relaxed, neutral position by the sides.

Stop the Five Seasons (continued)

Breathing In:

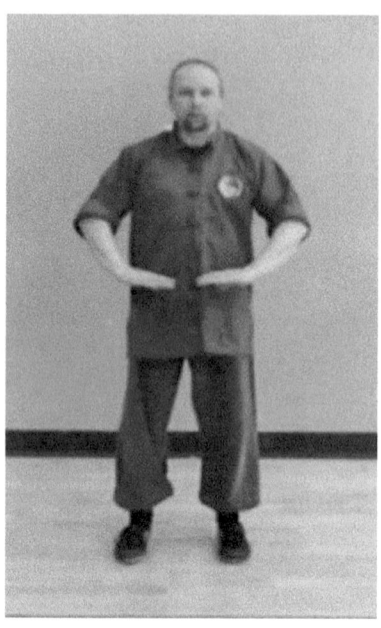

Posture: The hands circle up and inwards to finish with the palms down, fingertips pointing towards fingertips in front of the Lower Tantien.

Stop the Five Seasons (continued)

Breathing Out:

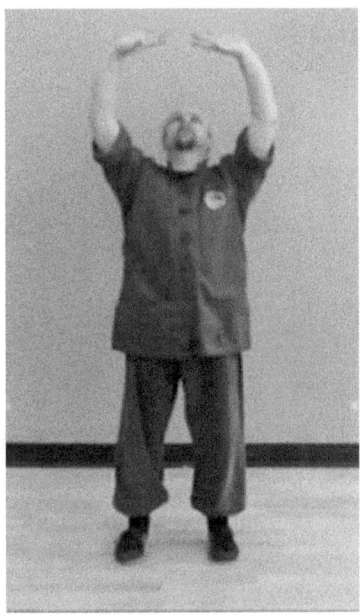

Posture: The hands come up in front of the body (with the palms facing away) until the palms are facing upwards above the head. As the hands come above the head, follow with the head until looking upwards.

Stop the Five Seasons (continued)

Breathing In:

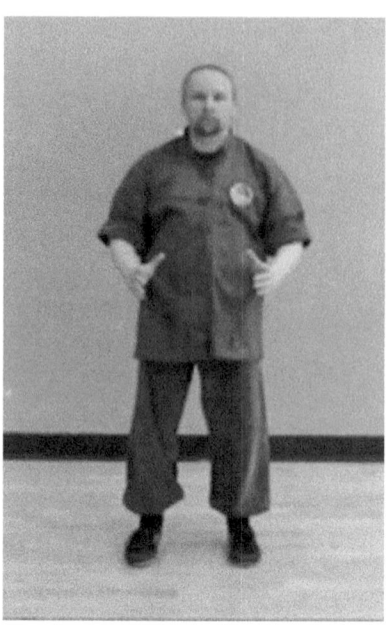

Posture: The hands reverse their movement to come down to finish in front of the abdomen as if holding a 'ball'. As the hands come down, the head returns to neutral.

Stop the Five Seasons (continued)

Breathing Out:

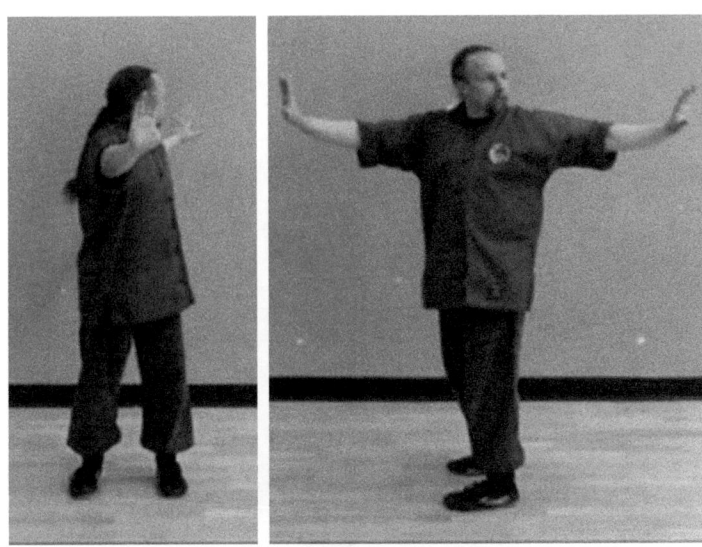

Posture: The right hand 'pushes' forwards and out to finish at shoulder height with the palm facing forwards. The left hand pushes out to shoulder height to the back (turning at the waist) and the head turns to look towards the left hand.

<u>Stop the Five Seasons</u> (continued)

Breathing In:

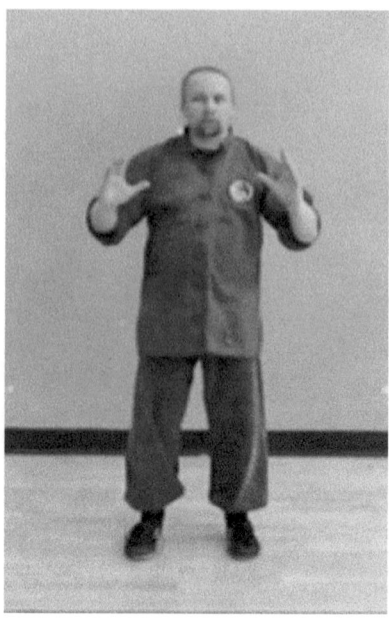

Posture: The hands reverse their movement to finish in front of the chest as if holding a 'ball'. The body turns back to face the front and the head returns to neutral.

Stop the Five Seasons (continued)

Breathing Out:

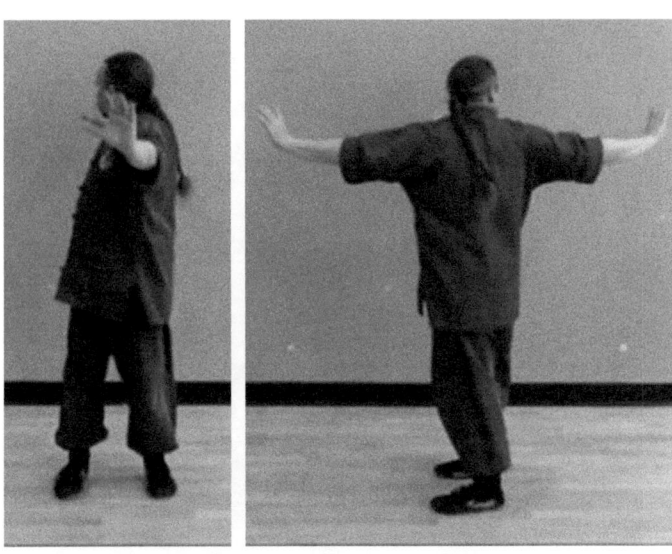

Posture: The left hand 'pushes' forwards and out to finish at shoulder height with the palm facing forwards. The right hand pushes out to shoulder height to the back (turning at the waist) and the head turns to look towards the right hand.

Stop the Five Seasons (continued)

Breathing In:

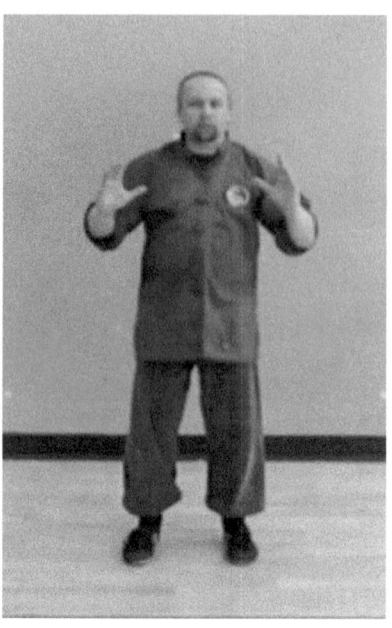

Posture: The hands reverse their movement to finish in front of the chest as if holding a 'ball'. The body turns back to face the front and the head returns to neutral.

Stop the Five Seasons (continued)

Breathing Out:

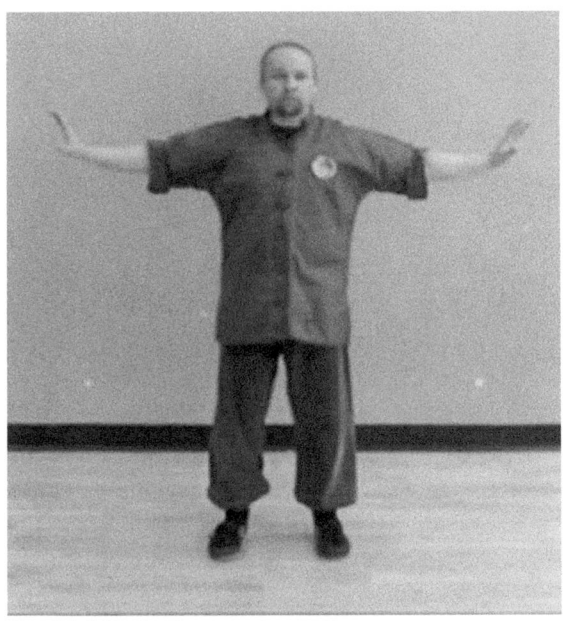

Posture: Both hands 'press' outwards to the sides at shoulder height. The head remains in a neutral position.

Stop the Five Seasons (continued)

Breathing In:

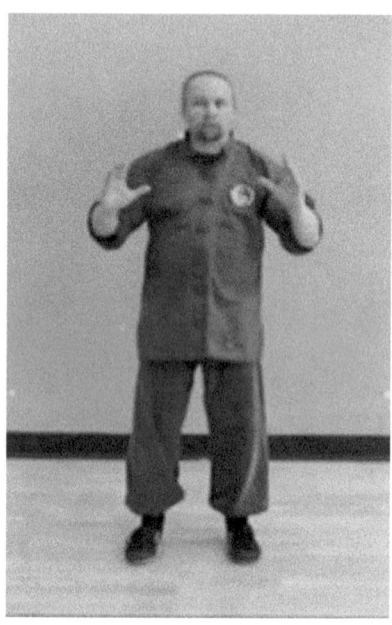

Posture: Draw the hands back in to a position as if holding a 'ball' in front of the chest.

Stop the Five Seasons (continued)

Breathing Out:

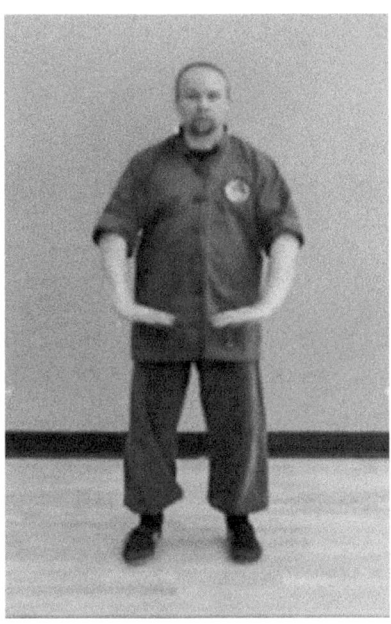

Posture: The hands press down in front of the body with the palms facing downwards (fingertips towards fingertips) until they are below Tantien height.

Stop the Five Seasons (continued)

Breathing In:

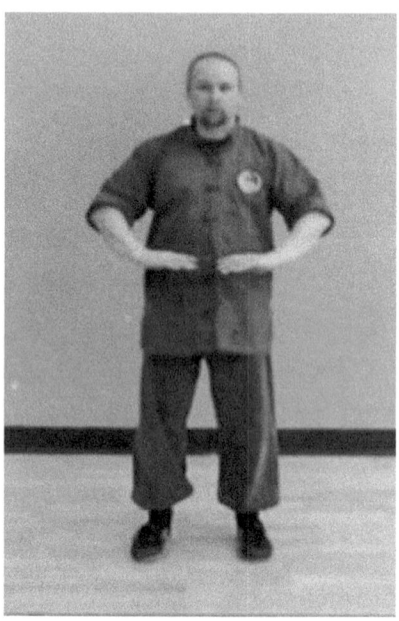

Posture: The hands raise in front of the body (still palms down and fingertips towards fingertips) until they are above the Tantien (ensure they are above navel height).

Stop the Five Seasons (continued)

Breathing Out:

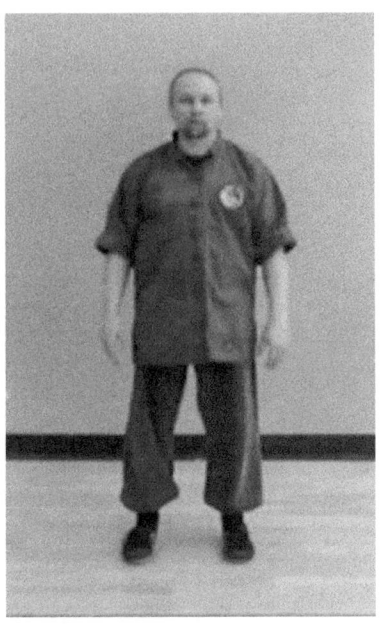

Posture: The hands lower to the sides into a neutral, relaxed position.

Notes: Repeat the entire exercise until you have done 4 or 8 repetitions.

Support the Clouds

Benefits: Heart

Start Position:

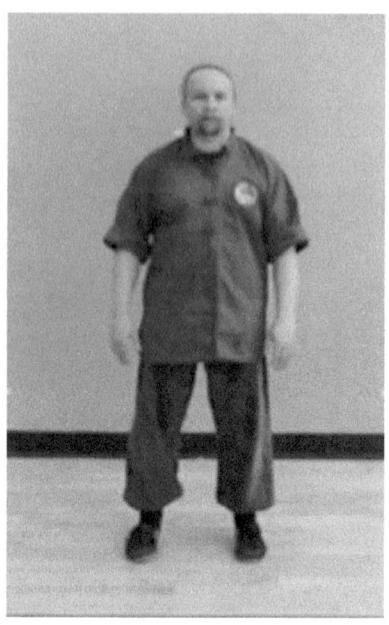

Stance: Remain in Bear stance throughout this exercise.
Posture: Arms start in a relaxed, neutral position by the sides.

Support the Clouds (continued)

Breathing In:

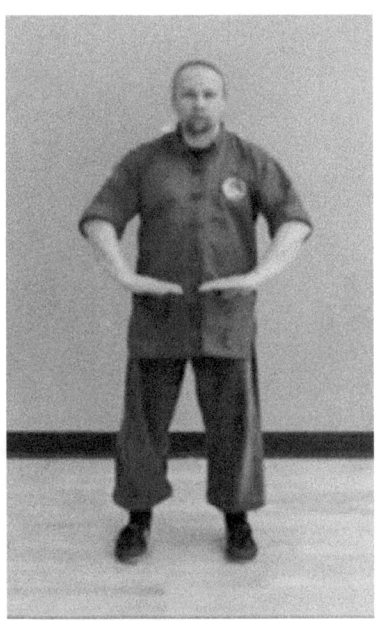

Posture: Both hands circle up and inwards to a position in front of the abdomen (Lower Tantien height) with the palms down and fingertips towards fingertips.

Support the Clouds (continued)

Breathing Out:

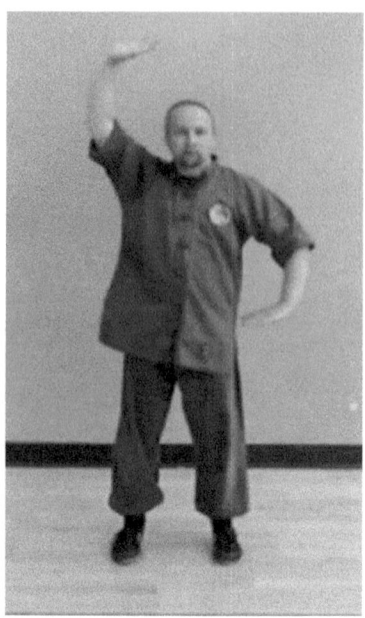

Posture: The right hand circles up in front of the body (palm faces away from the body) until the palm is upwards above the head. The left hand lowers to the side (palm still downwards) until the fingertips are pointing towards the hip. Note that both hands should finish their movements at the same time.

Support the Clouds (continued)

Breathing In:

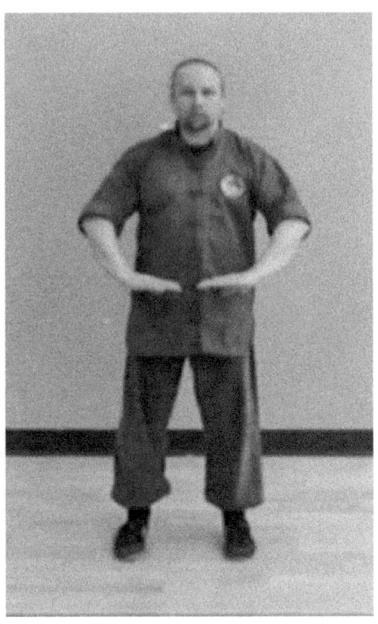

Posture: Both hands return to palms down, fingertips towards fingertips in front of the abdomen. Again, both hands should finish their movements at the same time.

Support the Clouds (continued)

Breathing Out:

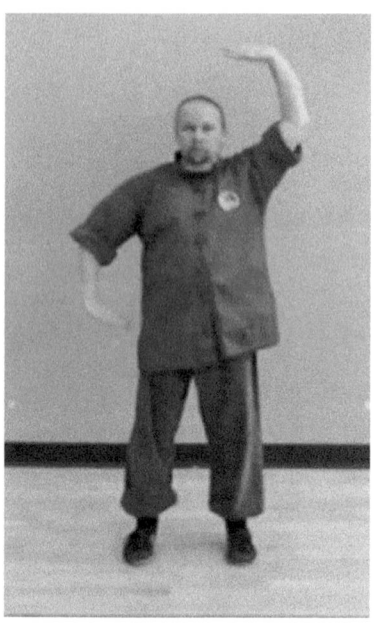

Posture: The left hand circles up in front of the body (palm faces away from the body) until the palm is upwards above the head. The right hand lowers to the side (palm still downwards) until the fingertips are pointing towards the hip. Note that both hands should finish their movements at the same time.

Support the Clouds (continued)

Breathing In:

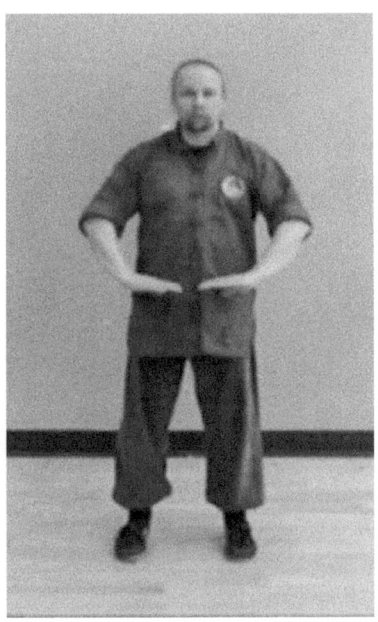

Posture: Both hands return to palms down, fingertips towards fingertips in front of the abdomen. Again, both hands should finish their movements at the same time.

Notes: Repeat the pattern until you have completed 8 repetitions.

Support the Clouds (continued)

Breathing Out:

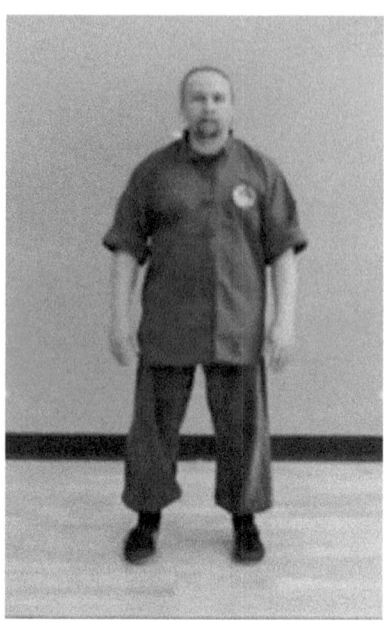

Posture: Lower the hands to the sides to a relaxed, neutral position.

Notes: Ensure that the elbow of the hand going downwards does not 'stick out' to the rear, but remains in the same plane as the body.

Section Three:

Stances.

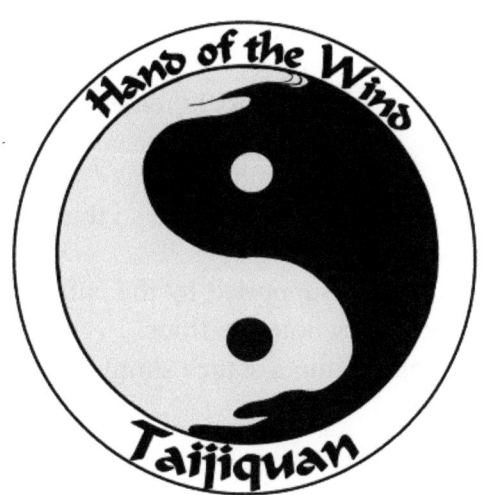

Stances.

General notes for all stances.

In Hand of the Wind Taijiquan and Qigong we use the term 'stance' to refer to the alignment of the lower body. Stance refers to alignment of the body from the waist down and we use 'posture' to refer to the alignment of the upper body, from the waist up (including arms, hands and head).

In all stances the basic principles must be adhered to, as taught within Hand of the Wind classes.

Key points to remember are:

- Never lock a limb.
- Pelvis should be aligned so that the tailbone is tucked underneath the body.
- Weight is supported by the ball of the foot.
- Toes relax onto the floor.
- Stepping into a stance should be heel-toe.

Within this section photographs are presented showing stances used within Taoyin exercises and the Taiji Form. For most of the stances there are also 'footprints' showing the correct foot placement and weight distribution – a black footprint shows a 'weighted' foot, a white footprint shows a foot with little or no weight in it and a grey footprint shows a foot supporting 50% of the body weight.

Eagle Stance.

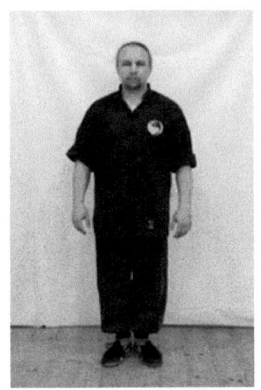
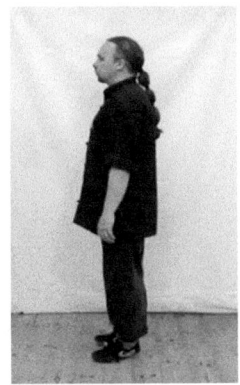

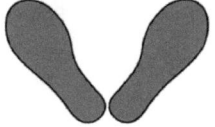

In Eagle stance the heels are together, the legs are straight (but not locked at the knees). The feet angle outwards from the centre line so that there is a maximum angle between the feet of 90° (although less than 90° is more relaxed for most people). The posture is maintained according to the basic principles and the weight is equally distributed between the feet.

Bear Stance.

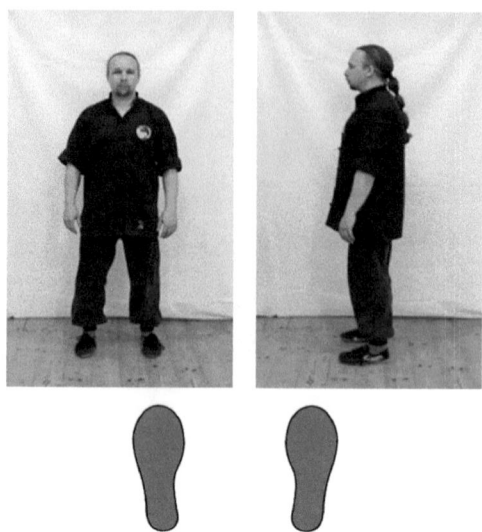

In Bear stance the feet are shoulder-width apart with the feet parallel, both pointing forwards. The knees are 'off-lock' so the legs are a little more bent than in Eagle stance but still with only a minimum amount of bend at the knees. Weight is evenly balanced on both feet.

Riding Horse Stance.

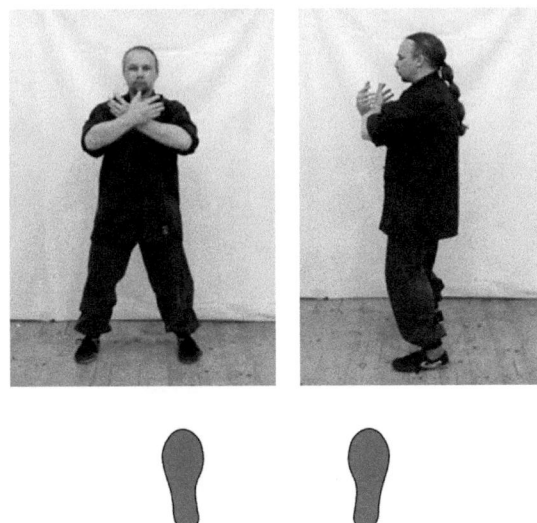

In Riding Horse the feet are wider than shoulder width, with the feet parallel so that the toes are pointing towards the front. The knees are more bent than in Bear stance so the feeling is that you are 'sitting' into the stance. The weight is equally distributed between both feet.

Leopard Stance.

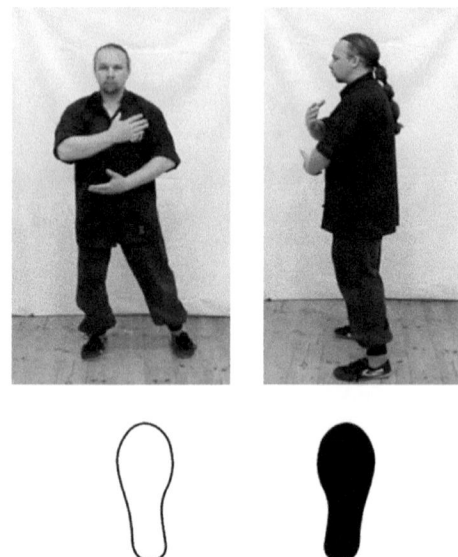

In Leopard the feet are at least shoulder width apart and parallel so the toes are pointing forwards. The weight is directed down into one foot with the knee of the weighted foot bent. The 'light' leg is straight (but not locked) with only the weight of the leg supported by that foot – the majority of the body-weight is supported by the bent leg.

Dragon Stance.

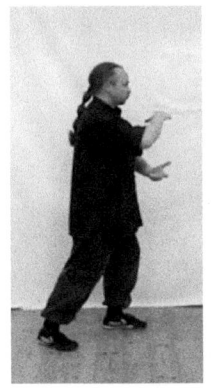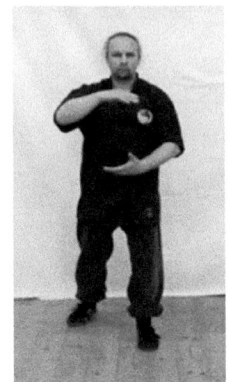

In Dragon the feet are shoulder width apart with one foot advanced to the front. Around 80% of the weight is supported on the front foot which is pointing forwards. The back foot is directed outwards on an angle similar to that in Eagle stance with little more than the weight of the back leg supported by that foot. The front leg is bent and the back leg is straight (but not locked and maintaining the pelvis alignment according to the basic principles). The weight is forward to almost the point where the back heel starts to lift, but not quite, so that the back foot remains flat on the ground. the hips are 'square' facing to the front and the front knee is not extended beyond the toes of the front foot.

Duck Stance.

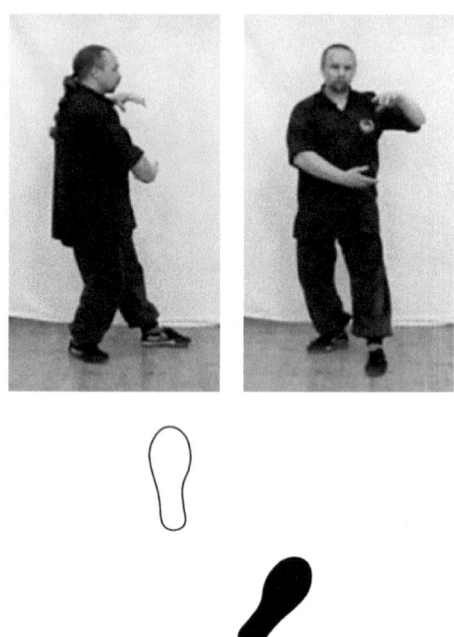

For Duck stance, the feet are shoulder width apart with the front foot pointing forwards and the back foot at an angle. The weight is in the back foot with only the weight of the front leg supported by the front foot. The rear knee is bent with the front leg straight, but not locked. Both feet are flat on the ground. The hips are 'square' facing to the front.

Crane Stance.

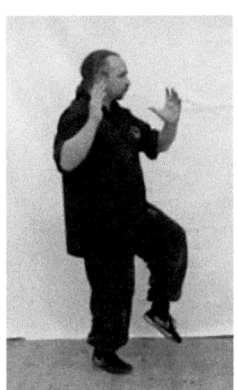 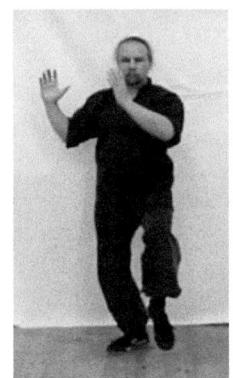

In Crane stance the front foot is lifted off the floor so that all the weight is supported by one foot which is aligned at an angle as in Eagle stance. The front knee is lifted to no higher than would bring the thigh parallel to the floor and the lower leg 'hangs' relaxed from the knee. The front foot relaxes down from the ankle maintaining the feeling of heel-toe as you 'step' into the stance. The standing (weighted) leg is bent at the knee.

Dog Stance.

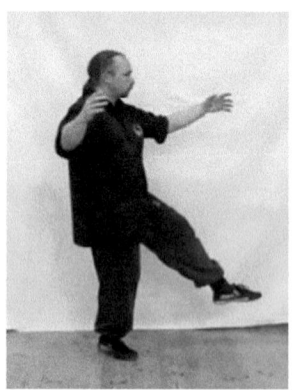 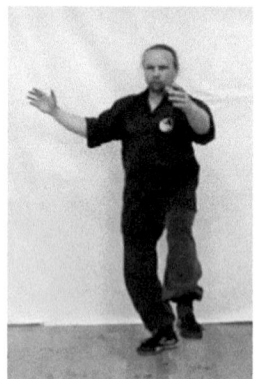

Dog stance is similar to Crane in that it is another stance where the front foot is lifted off the floor. In Dog stance the front foot is extended further forwards than the knee and again relaxes down from the ankle to 'step' heel-toe into the stance. The standing leg is bent and the front leg should be 'off-lock' and at a maximum height of thigh parallel to the floor.

Section Four:

Index of Taoyin Exercises.

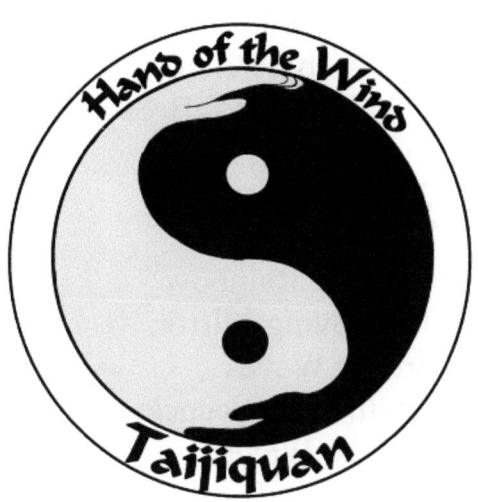

Alphabetical Index of Taoyin Exercises:

The Archer Turns Around	p19
Bend and Twist	p26
The Dragon Spits Fire	p37
Expand the Chest	p44
The Flying Fox	p47
Fly like the Dove	p52
Fly like the Wild Goose	p57
Four Directional Breathing	p64
The Growing Pine	p77
Happy Day	p80
Horsemanship	p85
Move the Rainbow	p89
The Moving Mirror	p96
Part the Waves	p107
Play the Shuttlecock	p115
Push the Wave	p128
Rock the Ball	p137
Rotate the Wheel	p140
Separate the Clouds	p145
Shao Gong (Large)	p148
Shao Gong (Small)	p151
Step Forwards and Look Back	p154
Stop the Five Seasons	p161
Support the Clouds	p174

Index of Taoyin Exercises classified by their benefits:

Balancing Qigong:

Four Directional Breathing	p64
Shao Gong (Large)	p148
Shao Gong (Small)	p151
Stop the Five Seasons	p161

Heart

The Archer Turns Around	p19
Fly like the Wild Goose	p57
Happy Day	p80
Horsemanship	p85
Part the Waves	p107
Separate the Clouds — best for heart	p145
Support the Clouds	p174

(handwritten annotations: "HP" next to Separate the Clouds; "HT" next to Support the Clouds)

Liver

Bend and Twist	p26
The Dragon Spits Fire	p37
Move the Rainbow	p89
The Moving Mirror	p96
Play the Shuttlecock	p115
Rotate the Wheel	p140
Step Forwards and Look Back	p154

(handwritten "L" next to The Dragon Spits Fire)

Lungs

The Archer Turns Around	p19
Expand the Chest	p44
The Flying Fox	p47
Fly like the Dove	p52

Spleen

Bend and Twist	p26
The Dragon Spits Fire	p37
Move the Rainbow	p89
The Moving Mirror	p96
Play the Shuttlecock	p115
Rotate the Wheel	p140
Step Forwards and Look Back	p154

Kidneys

Bend and Twist	p26
The Flying Fox	p47
The Growing Pine	p77
The Moving Mirror	p96
Part the Waves	p107
Play the Shuttlecock	p115
Push the Wave	p128
Rock the Ball	p137
Rotate the Wheel	p140
Step Forwards and Look Back	p154

Afterword:
A comment from the author.

    Qigong has been an integral part of my life for over twenty years and I have gained considerable benefits from my practice. I hope that this book will help you to gain more from your own practice of Qigong. Qigong is a huge field to study and there is a lot of information freely available now through the internet and the many published books on the subject. It is, without doubt, easier to find information now than it was when I began my studies of Qigong. However, this does increase the need to be discriminating in your studies and to consult an experienced teacher to gain the maximum benefits from your own practice.
    I wish you well with your Qigong and I hope it brings you as much pleasure and as many benefits as it has brought me over the years.
    Conrad Robinson, 2018.

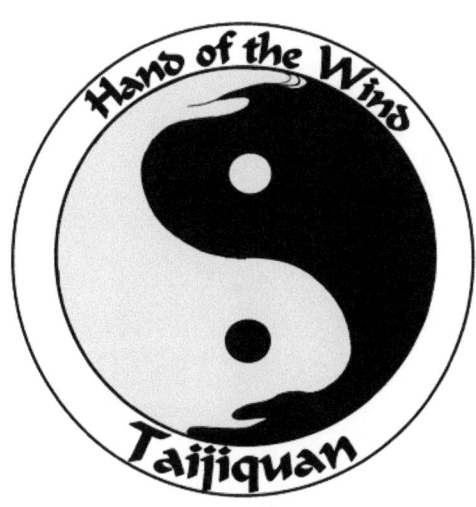

- Is the breath creating the movement or the movement creating the breath?
- For each movement – is the **benefit** of the stretch – does it out weigh the harm of the tension.
- Every movement is a realignment of the body – areas tense up to hold new position and relax to let other tensions go to take a new alignment due to movement
- The difference of breathing in or out on a portion of the exercise will affect what is stretched or worked. Be mindful of how the in or out breath affects the exercise and works entirely different things
- 3 sive and 12 sive breathing
  - split each 3 stre u.b 4 → 2 @ back, 2 @ front → feel the breathy
  relax breathing – do not tense abdominals to get a bigger breath. Tension restricts breath

Notes:

Notes:

Notes

Other exercises

Unsteady Rider → (Kidney)
Embrace knee to chest → (Liver) (joints + tendons)
Homage to the Stars → (Kidney)
Peace - Wic

Chicken & Vegetable Soup

1 packet chicken noodle soup   Water
1 each, grated: onion, turnip, carrot

Prepare chicken noodle soup as directed on packet; add vegetables then cook 15 minutes or until tender.

Creamy Carrot Soup

4 medium carrots, sliced   1 onion, sliced
30g butter, melted   Parsley, chopped
1/4 cup cream OR evaporated milk   Cayenne pepper
3 cups chicken stock OR water   Salt

In saucepan, add carrots & onion to butter; cook until soft. Add chicken stock or water; simmer 10 minutes then puree in blender. Return soup to pan with remaining stock; warm on low heat, add salt & pepper to taste.
Swirl in cream, sprinkle parsley over.

Beef & Vegetable Soup

1 shin beef   1 swede
2 large onions   2 potatoes
2 carrots   1 cup split peas OR soup mix
1 cup peas   Salt & pepper to taste

Put beef, onion, split peas, salt & pepper in boiler; boil until meat is leaving bone. Remove meat & bones then skim top of soup. Add all other vegetables; boil at least 1 hour adding more water as needed. Stir occasionally to prevent peas sticking to bottom of pot. Soup is better when re-heated.
Remove meat from bone and place in soup if liked. If not, remove meat from bone, chop, then put in flat bottom basin. Take 1 cup hot soup, add 1 dessertspoon gelatine; stir until dissolved then add to meat. Press down well then chill to set. Slice to use as sandwich meat or with salad.

Savoury Spread

1 teaspoon chopped onion
1/2 teaspoon curry powder
Parsley or spring onion tops
1 egg, hard boiled, chopped
Salt & pepper

Mix ingredients together then place on biscuits.

Sausage Savouries

500g mince or sausage meat
1 green apple, grated
1 tablespoon tomato sauce
1 teaspoon curry
2 teaspoons chutney
1 onion, chopped

Mix all ingredients together. Spread evenly over sheets of puff pastry; roll up then cut into 1/2" (125mm) wheels. Bake in moderate oven 25 minutes. Good hot or cold.

Leila's Fried Rice

Melt butter in frypan. Add chopped onion, chopped bacon, diced capsicum then toss & stir until onion tender. Beat 2 eggs, pour over top. Turn down heat; cover until eggs cooked then remove omelette; cut into small strips. To same pan add cold boiled rice, chicken cube, egg strips, salt & pepper. Stir. Cover, simmer until heated through.

Cheese Pie

1-1/2 cups grated cheese
2-1/2 cups milk
Bread & butter
2 eggs
Salt & pepper

Grease pie dish, then place alternate layers bread & butter with grated cheese until 3/4 full.
Beat eggs, milk, salt & pepper; pour over bread, allow to stand 30 minutes before baking in moderate oven 20 to 25 minutes or until knife placed in centre comes out clean.

Potato Pastry for Savoury Pies

1/2 cup mashed potato, creamy
1/4 cup dripping or butter
1 cup S.R. flour
1/2 teaspoon salt

Rub butter into flour & salt until like fine breadcrumbs. Mix in potato until well combined; use little water if needed; roll out. Use instead of any other pastry for savoury pie recipes.

Savoury Mince

500g mince
1 onion, chopped
1 teaspoon Worcestershire
1 tablespoon tomato sauce
1 carrot, grated
1 apple, grated
1 teaspoon curry powder

Place all in saucepan and simmer 20 minutes. Serve on bed of white rice.

Savoury BBQ Chops or Steak

Place number of chops and/or steaks required on oven tray; sprinkle with french onion soup. Cover tray completely with foil, then place in centre of cold oven. Turn oven to 350°C (180°F) then cook 1 hour.

Potato Cakes

Bacon scraps
Salt & pepper
60g plain flour
250g mashed potato
Pinch mixed herbs

Fry bacon, chop finely. Mix all together, shape into small cakes 1/2" (12mm) thick on floured board. Fry in pan until golden brown.

Macaroni & Cheese

Boil 3/4 cup macaroni in salted water. Make white sauce. Fill buttered ovenproof dish with layers of macaroni, white sauce & grated cheese. Place in moderate oven to brown.

Noodle Omelette

1 packet 2 minute noodles   2 eggs
1 tablespoon butter

    Place noodles in saucepan with 1 cup water (reserve spice sachet); boil 2 minutes then drain.
    Beat eggs with spice sachet. Heat butter in pan, mix noodles with eggs then tip quickly into hot pan; cook until underside is golden brown. Turn omelette over to cook 2nd side. Serve immediately with salad or cold meat.

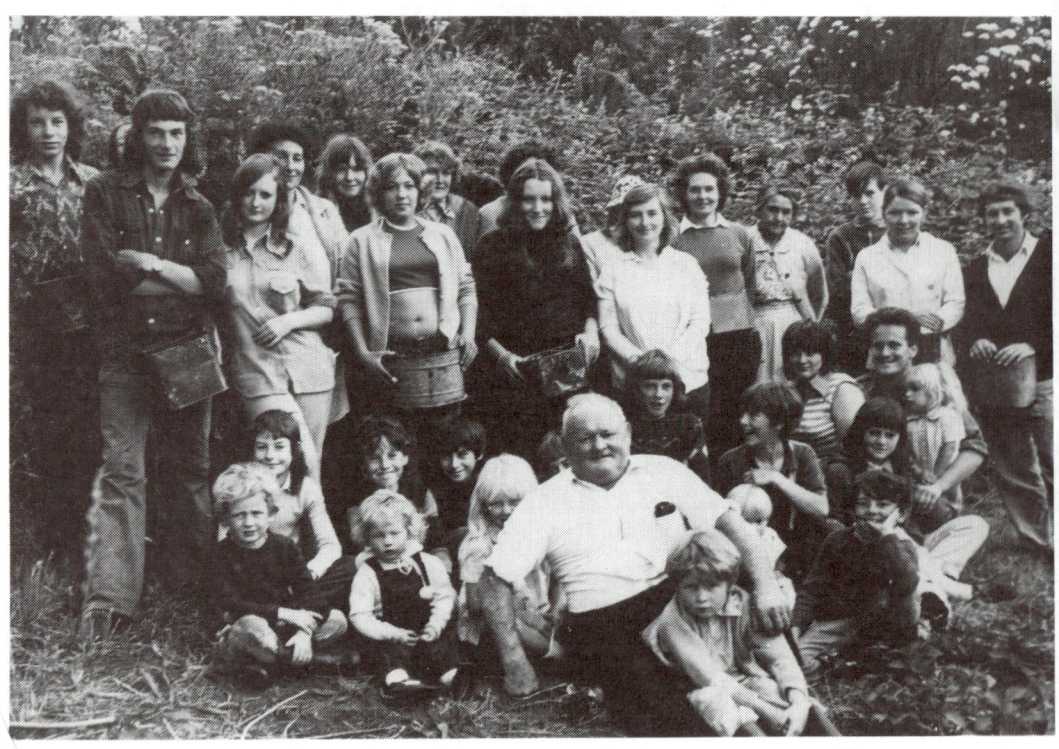

Family and pickers pose at the Franklin farm.

Rice Salad

    1 cup rice, cook until tender. Pour on french dressing while hot. When cool add:
- 1/4 small onion, chopped
- 1/4 cup peas
- 1/2 cup ham, chopped
- 1/4 capsicum, chopped
- 1/4 cup corn

Chill and serve.

Italian Mushroom Salad

500g button mushrooms
1 small bottle Italian dressing
2 teaspoons parsley, chopped
1 green capsicum
1 red capsicum
1 large onion

Slice mushrooms, onions & capsicum into rounds finely as possible; mix with parsley, then chill. Just before serving, pour dressing over, mix well.

Crunchy Salad

1 small apple, diced
1/4 cup almonds, finely chopped
2 eggs, hard boiled, sliced
Juice 1 lemon

1 cup each: Cucumber, diced   Celery, diced
Shallots, sliced   Rice, cooked

Toss apple in lemon juice to prevent browning. Mix together apple, almonds, rice & vegetables, then mix salad dressing through; garnish with egg.

Apple Salad

2 green apples
Juice 1/4 lemon
4 tablespoons chopped nuts
125g diced tasty cheese
2 red apples
Grated carrot
French dressing

Core then dice unpeeled apples; sprinkle with lemon juice. Add other ingredients then toss lightly.

Potato Salad

5 medium potatoes, cooked, diced
1 tablespoon prepared mustard
1/4 cup chopped parsley
Radishes, sliced
Salad dressing
1/2 cup diced celery
2 eggs, hard boiled
1/4 cup diced onion
Fresh lettuce

Mix onion, parsley, celery & potatoes; season to taste. Chop eggs; mix with dressing & mustard; add to potato mixture. Place in bowl lined with lettuce then garnish with radish.

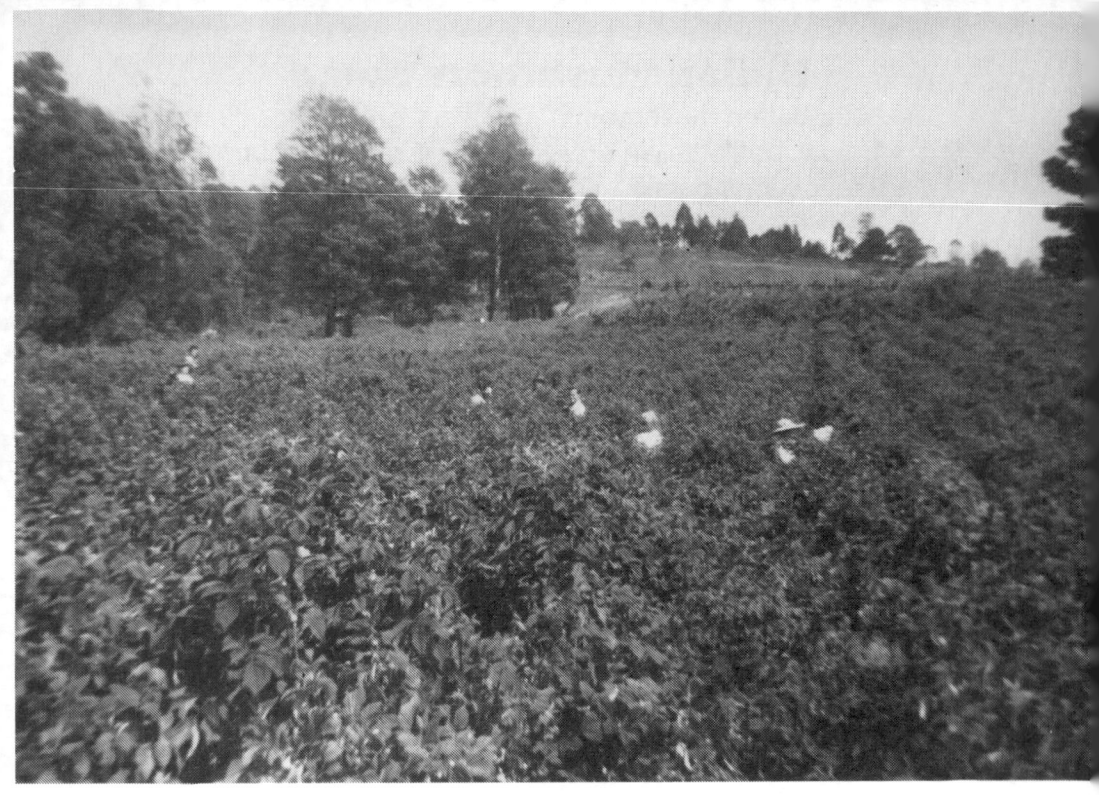

Picking raspberries in the Huon.

Salad Dressing (1)

1 dessertspoon butter
1/2 teaspoon mustard
1 teaspoon sugar
3 tablespoons vinegar
1/2 teaspoon salt
1 egg
6 tablespoons milk

Melt butter in saucepan, add salt, sugar & mustard. Mix well, add egg, beat well. Add milk then vinegar; cook until thick. DO NOT BOIL

Salad Dressing (2)

Beat together: 2 eggs, 1 teaspoon salt,
1 teaspoon mustard, 1 tin sweetened condensed milk.

Add 1 cup vinegar little at a time, beating well. Store in refrigerator in screw top jar. Keeps for weeks. Add milk or cream to thin.

The Huon Valley must be one of the few places on earth where you can really adapt your cooking skills to match a limited or high budget, and live extremely well at either end of the scale. We have a climate that allows us to have an abundance of fruit and vegetables. Water is so close at all points that we have access to a wide variety of sea food.

Many of the seafood recipes in this book have come about from holidaying at Southport with my family, we would spend days fishing for flathead or walking on the rocks collecting oysters, and the nights fishing for flounder. Between times the boys with their father would dive for abalone. When you became tired of eating fish one way, you invented another way of cooking it.

Quick Abalone (1)

Trim, slice and bash abalone. Heat BBQ, place little oil on plate. Place abalone on plate, turn almost immediately, cook other side, taking no more than one minute or meat will toughen.

Quick Abalone (2)

Trim, slice and bash abalone; dip in beaten egg then into breadcrumbs. Place in hot oil or butter, turn quickly; remove from pan.

Abalone tends to spit badly if overcooked, so if using oil, take care.

Any fish is suitable to wrap in foil and cook on BBQ. It keeps its flavour and juices. Do not overcook or it will dry out. A variety of fruit and vegetables can be included in the foil with the fish.

Baked Trevalla or Trevally

Place fillets of fish on greased tray; cook in moderate oven about 15 minutes. Remove from oven, sprinkle lemon juice & pepper over, then cover with grated cheese. Return to oven for 5 minutes.

Baked Atlantic Salmon

Leave fish whole; fill body cavity with zucchini, tomato, onion, salt & pepper. Place fish on foil, smear with little butter, sprinkle black pepper; cover with foil, folding all edges together. Bake in moderate oven 45 minutes to 1 hour.

When cooked skin will lift back with the foil, fish can be lifted from bone with spatula into individual serves.

Serve with seafood sauce:

    1/4 cup cream   1/4 cup mayonnaise
    1/4 cup tomato sauce   1/4 teaspoon black pepper

Beat well, chill.

Salmon Pate

250g Philadelphia cream cheese   Chives, chopped
500g salmon   Parsley, chopped
1 cup mayonnaise   Salt & pepper
125g melted butter   2 Tablespoons lemon juice

Add cheese to butter and blend. Add all other ingredients and blend until smooth. Can be frozen.

Quick Cheese & Salmon

90g grated cheese   250g salmon (or any fish)
1 cup raw rice   2 teaspoons Worcestershire
1/2 onion, chopped   Salt & pepper
Parsley

Flake fish with fork. Cook rice then drain well. Melt butter, add rice & fish; season to taste. Stir in 60g cheese & onion then heat well. Garnish with rest of cheese & parsley.

Mock Scallops

1kg flathead fillets   3 cups milk
2 tablespoons flour   Salt & pepper
1 tablespoon curry powder

Bring milk to boil, thicken with dry ingredients mixed with little milk. Drop in diced flathead then cook until meat is white; serve immediately.

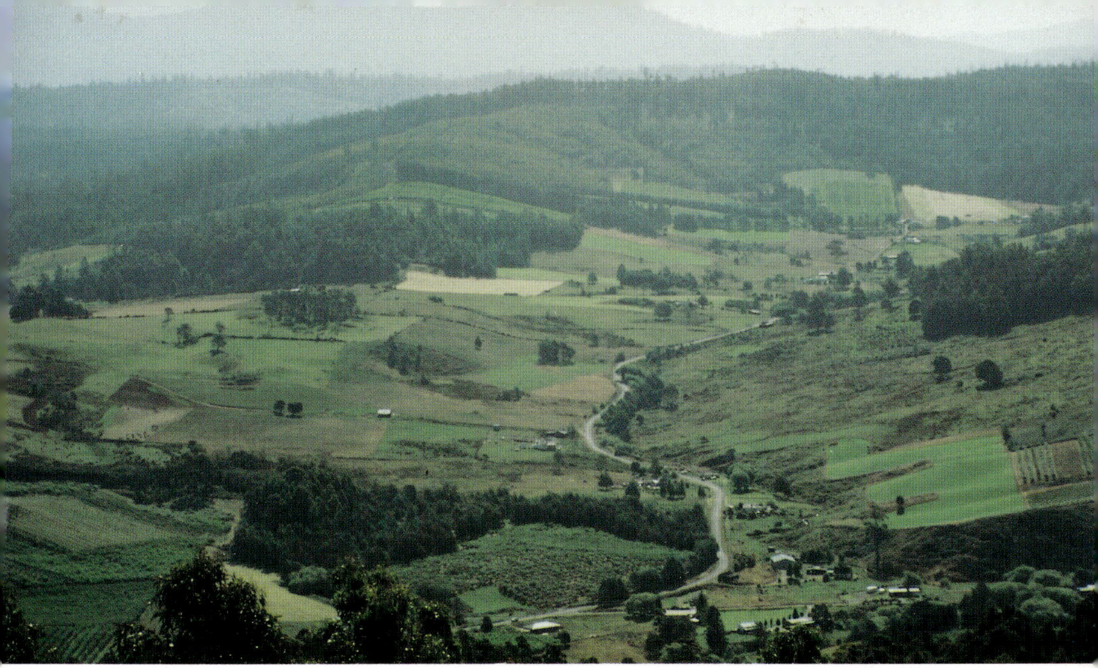

Four Foot Road winds down from the hills to Geeveston; on the original 4' tramway made from saplings, trains carried logs to the sawmill.

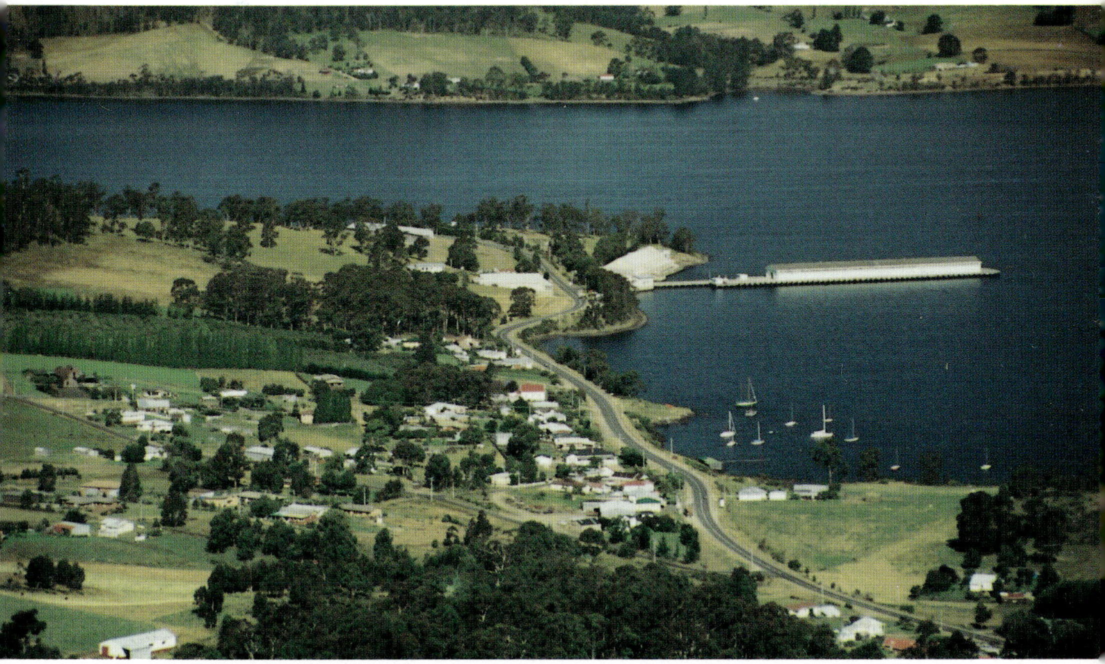

From the Port Huon wharf many ships have loaded fruit and timber for world wide destinations. Modern techniques have led to its disuse. The Huon waterways are a yachting paradise.

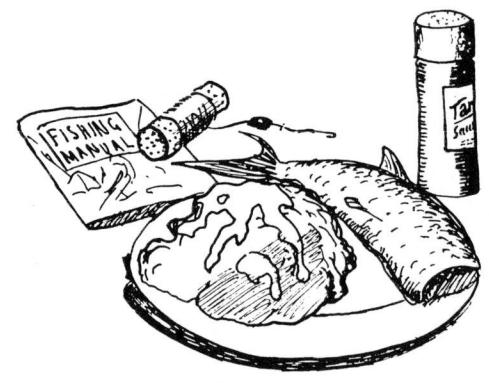

Abalone Patties

500g abalone
3 rashers bacon
Parsley
1 cup mashed potato
1 onion
Salt & pepper

Mince abalone, bacon & onion. Mix with potato, parsley, salt & pepper. Form into small balls, flatten out then coat with flour. Fry in hot oil until brown both sides. Can BBQ. Avoid over cooking.

Battered Cod Fillets

Fillet fish, coat with plain flour. Then dip in batter.
Batter: 1 cup plain flour   1 cup beer
Salt & pepper to taste

Place flour, salt & pepper in bowl; make well in centre, add beer slowly, beating well. Allow to stand few minutes. Heat oil in pan until faint smoke rises, place fish in oil, cook quickly both sides.

Easy Fish Dish

1 can salmon
1 can peas
1 pkt chicken noodle soup
Tasty cheese, grated
Fresh bread crumbs
1 can corn kernels
1 cup rice
1 dessertspoon curry powder
Medium white sauce

Boil rice with soup, drain then add fish, corn, peas & curry. Mix then place in ovenproof dish. Top with white sauce & breadcrumbs; cover with grated cheese. Place in moderate oven until brown.

Seafood Supreme
Microwave
Crayfish, Scallops, Prawns or Crab

2 tablespoons butter	1 cup: 1/2 milk, 1/2 cream
2 tablespoons flour	1/2 cup milk
1/2 teaspoon salt	2 egg yolks, beaten
1/4 teaspoon paprika	Dash pepper

Place butter in casserole dish, micro until melted. Stir in flour, paprika, salt & pepper. Blend in milk & cream mix, then remaining milk; micro on High until thick, 4 to 7 minutes. Stir 2 or 3 times during cooking.

Stir small amount hot sauce into egg yolk, then add to casserole. Micro on high until thick, 1 to 3 minutes.

Stir in desired fish then micro on High 1 to 3 minutes.

Port Huon Scallop Pie

500g scallops	1 dessertspoon butter
1 tablespoon flour	1/2 teaspoon dry mustard
1 teaspoon curry powder	1/4 teaspoon salt
1 cup milk	1 teaspoon Worcestershire
Squeeze lemon juice (optional)	1/2 cup breadcrumbs

Wash scallops well then drain. Place in greased ovenproof dish.

Melt butter, cover with half breadcrumbs, add flour, mustard, curry & salt. Stir 2 to 3 minutes over low heat; add milk, stir until boiling. Carefully fold in sauce & lemon juice; pour over scallops. Sprinkle remaining breadcrumbs, dot with butter. Bake in moderate oven 15 to 20 minutes.

Cheesy Oysters

Place enough oysters (shelled) to cover bottom of 20cm pie plate. Chop 4 rashers bacon & 1/2 onion; place over oysters. Sprinkle 4 tablespoons Worcestershire sauce over then cover with grated cheese.

Place in very hot oven until cheese melts, about 5 minutes. Brown under grill; serve immediately.

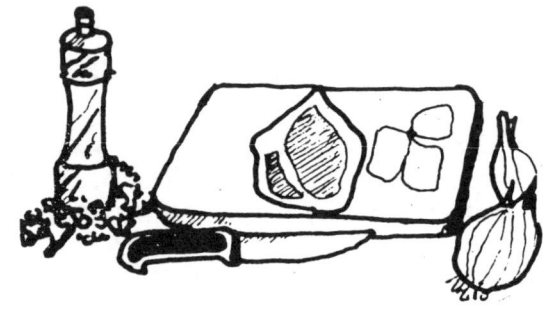

Savoury Steak

1kg blade steak
2 teaspoons sugar
1/2 teaspoon pepper
3 teaspoons Worcestershire
1-1/2 cups cold water

3 teaspoons flour
1/4 teaspoon mustard
1/2 teaspoon salt
4 tablespoons vinegar

Mix dry ingredients then coat steak; place in casserole dish. Mix together Worcestershire, vinegar & water; pour over steak. Cook in moderate oven until sauce begins to thicken, then cook in very slow oven 2 hours.

Sliced carrots & potatoes can be cooked on top.

Rabbit Patties

1 rabbit
2 rashers bacon
3/4 cup cold water
1 tablespoon cooking oil

1 onion
1 cup soft breadcrumbs
Salt to taste
Flour

Cut all meat from uncooked rabbit then put through mincer with other ingredients. Add water & salt; mix well together. Form into patties with little flour.

Put in ovenproof dish with hot oil then bake in moderate oven 3/4 hour. Serve with brown gravy.

Steak & Kidney Dumplings

1kg steak & kidney
1/2 cup peas
1 carrot, diced

1 large onion
1 potato, diced
Salt & pepper

Place all ingredients in saucepan then simmer until steak is tender. Avoid overcooking. Thicken lightly with flour & parisian essence mixed with little water.

Oxtail & Dumplings

Cooked in same way as Steak & Kidney. Substitute kangaroo tail if wished.

Mince & Dumplings

Cooked in same way as Steak & Kidney.

Dumplings

2 large cups S.R. flour	90g butter
Salt	1 egg
1/4 teaspoon mixed herbs (optional)	Water

Rub butter into flour with salt; add egg then mix with enough water to form soft dough. Form into balls (about 2 tablespoons of dough). Roll in flour, put on top of simmering meat. Cook about 15 minutes. Avoid lifting lid. Turn stove to lowest setting after adding thickening to meat.

Savoury Mince

500g mince	1 teaspoon curry powder
1/2 cup uncooked rice	4 rashers bacon
1 400g can vegetable soup	1 400g can water

Mix all ingredients except bacon together then place in greased ovenproof dish. Cook uncovered in moderate oven 1 to 1-1/4 hours; 15 minutes before taking out, place bacon rashers on top of mince to brown.

Sweet & Sour Pork

1 kg lean meat	1 onion
1/4 cup capsicums	1 carrot, chopped
1 large apple, chopped	1 cup pineapple pieces

Fry meat & onion until brown. Place in saucepan meat, onion & vegetables. Mix together:

2 dessertspoons brown sugar	1 cup pineapple juice
2 teaspoons vinegar	1 cup water
2 tablespoons soy sauce	

Pour over meat & vegetables then cook slowly 1/2 hour. Thicken with cornflour mixed to paste with water. Serve with rice.

Lambs Fry & Bacon

1 lambs fry
1 large onion, sliced
6 rashers bacon
Salt & pepper to taste
2 tablespoons plain flour
1/2 teaspoon parisian essence

Soak fry in salt water 1 hour, then skin, slice into strips, coat in flour then fry in little oil until brown. Remove fry then place bacon & onion in pan; when onion is soft remove from pan. Sprinkle flour into pan then cook adding water slowly until thickness required. Add parisian essence, salt, pepper, bacon, onion then fry and simmer 30 minutes.

Curried Rabbit

1 rabbit
2 large carrots, chopped
1 large onion, chopped
1 swede, chopped
1 tablespoon curry powder
2 tablespoons flour
Salt & pepper to taste
1 cup peas

Joint rabbit into 7 pieces (2 back legs, 2 front legs, body in three equal parts). Place meat in large saucepan with vegetables, salt & pepper, cover with water, then boil 1 hour or until rabbit is tender. Make paste of flour, curry powder & little water; add to meat then simmer 10 minutes. Serve with creamed potato, mashed pumpkin & beans.

Rabbit in Batter

1 rabbit, jointed
1 onion, chopped
1 egg
Little milk
Salt & pepper
1 cup S.R. flour
Pinch salt

Place rabbit, onion, salt & pepper in saucepan then cover with water; boil until meat is tender. Remove rabbit, allow to cool; reserve liquid for gravy. Mix flour, egg & pinch salt with enough milk to make batter consistency. Heat oil in large pan. Coat rabbit with plain flour, then dip in batter, place in pan, cook until golden brown, turning once. Make gravy by thickening liquid with plain flour & parisian essence, mixed to paste with water.

Casserole of Rabbit or Chicken

Cut 1 boiler fowl or rabbit into small pieces. Fry 1 sliced onion until golden brown; remove from pan. Dip pieces of meat into seasoned flour then fry in same pan until brown. Place in ovenproof dish with onion; add 300mls cream, 250g mushrooms, salt & pepper. Cover dish; cook in moderate oven 2 hours. If gravy needs thickening, add 1 tablespoon flour mixed with little water or milk.

Minted Lamb Chops

4 tablespoons fresh mint, chopped   1/2 cup cooking oil
1 large clove garlic, crushed   1/2 cup lemon juice
1/2 teaspoon finely chopped lemon rind   Salt & pepper

In flat ovenproof dish mix all ingredients. Add 6 lamb chops then marinade 4 hours. Grill chops both sides, basting with marinade. Serve with potatoes, minted peas & baby carrots.

Casseroled Stuffed Lamb Hearts

4 lamb hearts   60g dripping
1 rasher bacon, chopped   1 cup breadcrumbs
2 teaspoons chopped parsley   1/2 teaspoon mixed herbs
Salt to taste   Milk to bind

Mix all ingredients together and stuff hearts. Coat hearts in flour then fry until well browned. Remove from pan. Stir 1/2 cup plain flour into pan then cook 2 minutes. Slowly stir in 1 pint water then bring to boil, turn down heat, continue stirring until thickened.

Place hearts in casserole; add
         2 onions, sliced   3 carrots, sliced
         1 turnip, diced   Parsley, chopped

Pour gravy over then cook in moderate oven 1-1/2 hours or until vegetables & meat are tender.

Savoury Chops

6 large lamb leg chops   4 tablespoons tomato sauce
2 large onions, sliced   3 tablespoons Worcestershire
Salt & pepper

Place trimmed chops in large saucepan with onion, sauces and seasoning; cover with water then boil until tender. Thicken with paste of plain flour and water.

Lamb Spareribs in BBQ Sauce

1-1/2 kg breast of lamb
1 onion, chopped
1 clove garlic (optional)
3 tablespoons tomato sauce
1 teaspoon salt & pepper
Water
2 tablespoons brown vinegar
1 tablespoon Worcestershire
1 tablespoon chutney
1 tablespoon brown sugar
1 tablespoon chopped parsley

Cut lamb into ribs and place in fry pan or covered oven dish over low heat; cook until fat has rendered from meat. Remove meat then drain off fat from pan. Place all ingredients in pan with enough water to blend. Return meat to pan then simmer 45 minutes - 1 hour, adding more water as needed.

Braised Lamb Shanks

2 tablespoons cooking oil
1 carrot, diced
1/2 tablespoon sugar
1 onion, chopped
1 tablespoon Worcestershire
1 cup tomato pulp or 1 400g can
4 lamb shanks
1 stick celery
1 clove garlic
Parsley, chopped
Salt & pepper
5 tablespoons water

Heat oil, add shanks, then cook until brown. Remove shanks, drain pan; return pan to heat then add onion, garlic, carrot & celery. Cook 5 minutes then stir in tomatoes, salt, pepper, sugar, water & sauce. Return shanks to pan; cover then simmer 1-1/2 to 2 hours. Add more water if needed.

Sweet Curried Neck Chops

1 kg neck chops
1 onion, chopped
1 tablespoon curry powder
2 tablespoons brown sugar
1-1/2 tablespoons brown vinegar
1 apple, chopped
2 tablespoons flour
1/2 cup sultanas
3 cups water
Salt to taste

Trim chops of fat and place in saucepan with onion, apple & water. Cook until tender then add sultanas; mix all other ingredients to a paste with little water then add to chops to thicken. Simmer on very low heat 10 minutes. Serve with boiled rice, green beans & shoestring carrots.

Steamed Meat & Veg Pudding

Dice: 500g blade steak   2 carrots
             3 tomatoes   2 onions
Add: 2-1/2 cups water   1 dessertspoon parsley
            1/2 teaspoon salt   1/4 teaspoon pepper

Simmer until tender, strain off stock to keep. Leave meat & veg to cool.

Batter: 6 tablespoons S.R. flour   1 teaspoon butter
              1 egg   1/2 cup milk

Stir meat & veg into batter & mix well. Pour into greased steamer then cook 2 hours. Thicken stock to serve as gravy over pudding.

Liver & Veg Pie

1 liver, cut in thin strips   Sliced/shredded vegetables

Grease large ovenproof dish. Put layer of liver, then layers of sliced potato, carrot (or other root vegetable), onion, shredded cabbage. Continue until dish is filled. Pour in 1 cup water, dot with little butter. Bake in medium oven 1-1/2 hours.

Camp Pie

3 cups mince   1 cup fine breadcrumbs
1 cup bacon, minced   Salt & pepper
1 tablespoon Worcestershire   1 cup milk
1 teaspoon thyme or mixed herbs

Mix all ingredients together. Place in greased steamer then steam 2 hours. Allow to become cold before turning out.

Tripe

Make white sauce, flavour with 2 teaspoons curry. Simmer tripe in sauce 15 minutes.

Beat 2 egg yolks then stir into tripe. Place in ovenproof dish, cover with breadcrumbs, dot with butter, then brown quickly in hot oven.

Marinated Chicken Wings
(Microwave)

12 chicken wings
2 tablespoons soy sauce
1 tablespoon white vinegar
2 teaspoons lemon juice (opt)
2 tablespoons brown sugar
1 tablespoon Worcestershire
1/2 teaspoon ground ginger
1/4 cup water

Disjoint wings, discard tips. Arrange wings in dish, combine all other ingredients then micro on High 2 minutes. Pour hot marinade over wings, cover and stand at room temperature 3 to 4 hours, or overnight in refrigerator. Drain marinade, cover then micro 3-4 minutes on High. Let stand 3 minutes before serving.

Sausage Surprise
(Microwave)

500g thin beef sausages
2 teaspoons vinegar
1 tablespoon brown sugar
2 teaspoons Worcestershire
1 teaspoon dry mustard
3 tablespoons tomato sauce

Split sausages lengthways then place in dish. Mix all other ingredients together, pour over sausages. Cook on High 7-10 minutes.

Can be grilled; cook round side of sausages, turn split side up, pour over sauce then grill.

Mince Porcupines

500g mince
1/2 cup raw rice
1 cup water
1 can tomato soup*
1 onion, chopped
Salt & pepper

Grease casserole, mix mince, rice, onion, salt & pepper to form balls. Place in dish, pour over soup & water mixed together. Bake covered in moderate oven 1 hour.

* Thin brown gravy can be used instead of soup.

Pasta Bake

3 cups spiral noodles, cooked
1/2 cup bacon, chopped
1 packet cheese & leek soup
2-1/2 cups milk
2 tablespoons butter
3/4 cup grated cheese

Melt butter, add blended soup mix & milk; place on heat then stir until boiling. Combine with noodles & bacon. Pour into ovenproof dish, sprinkle cheese over; bake in moderate oven 15 to 20 minutes.

Farmhouse Beef Casserole

500g blade steak, cubed
2 cloves garlic, crushed
1 cup beef stock
1 large potato, cubed
1 large onion, chopped
1 cup mushrooms
2 bay leaves
1 cup celery
2 tomatoes, chopped

Place all ingredients in casserole with lid on and cook in moderate oven for 1-1/2 hours.

Can be microwaved - 10 minutes on High, then medium-low 45 minutes.

Potato Boats

(Microwave)

4 medium potatoes, scrubbed, pricked with fork
1/3 cup shredded cheese   1/4 cup onion, chopped
1/2 cup sour cream   1 teaspoon salt

Bake potatoes on high, 12 - 14 minutes. Blend cream, onion, cheese & salt. Slice top off each potato or cut in half through middle, then scrape out insides. Add potato to cheese mix and blend well. Stuff potato mix back into shells, then bake 1 minute on High before serving.

Vegetable Pie

Boil sufficient vegetables of your choice to fill casserole dish, making sure they are still a bit crunchy. Top with white sauce, breadcrumbs & grated cheese.

Bake in moderate oven 10-15 minutes.

Basic Family Meat Loaf

1kg mince
1 teaspoon salt
1 onion, chopped
1/4 teaspoon dry herbs
1 cup soft breadcrumbs
1 cup milk
Pepper
3 or 4 rashers bacon

Combine all ingredients except bacon. Place in dish; top with bacon. Bake in moderate oven 1 hour or until loaf shrinks from sides of pan.

Potato Mince Bake

500g mince
1 large onion, chopped
60g butter
30g flour
1 cup grated cheese
Salt & pepper
1/4 teaspoon mixed herbs
750g potatoes
1-1/4 cups milk

Fry onion in butter, add mince then cook until brown. Add salt, pepper & mixed herbs. Slice potatoes thinly. Place alternate layers of mince & potato in ovenproof dish, finishing with potato.

Melt 30g butter, stir in flour, add milk gradually; bring to boil; cook 3 minutes then stir in cheese. Add salt & pepper. Pour sauce over potatoes then bake in moderate oven 1 hour or until tender and brown.

Wallaby Patties

1kg wallaby mince
500g beef mince
1 large onion, chopped
Salt & pepper
1/4 teaspoon mixed herbs
1/2 apple, grated
1 carrot, grated
1 egg
Parsley
2 tablespoons flour

Mix all ingredients together, adding flour last only if too wet to form firm balls. Make into balls using about 2 tablespoons for each. Coat with flour, flatten and fry or barbecue until cooked. Can be placed in ovenproof dish after cooking, covered with gravy and simmered in moderate oven for 30 minutes.

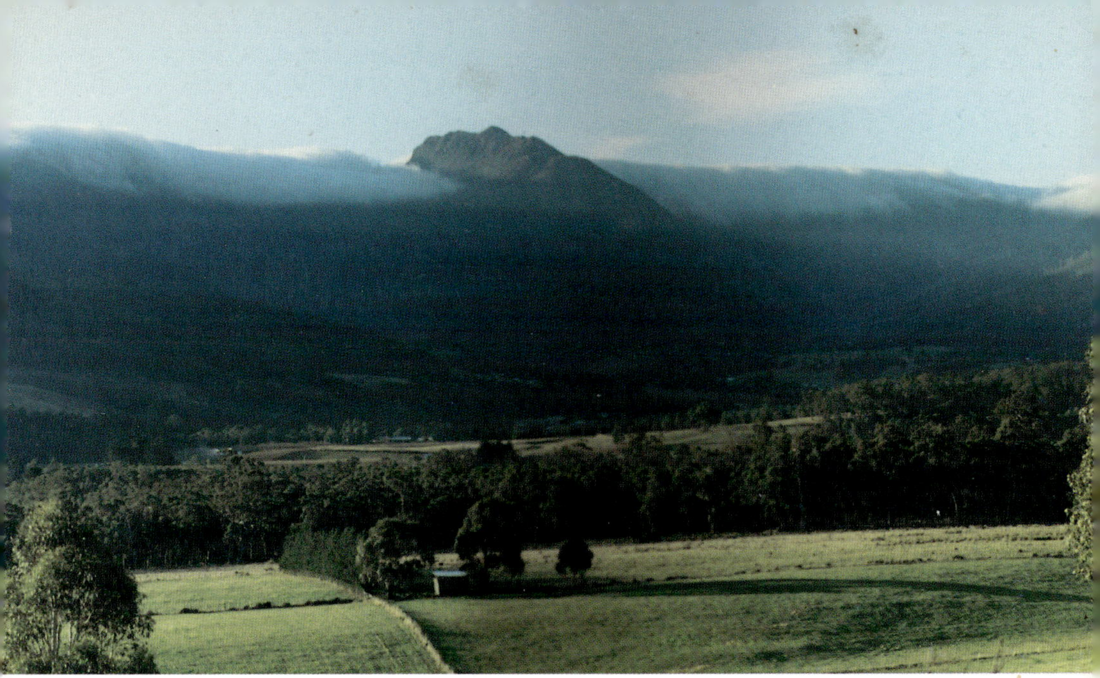

The Sleeping Beauty (Huon Belle) mountain dominates the valley.

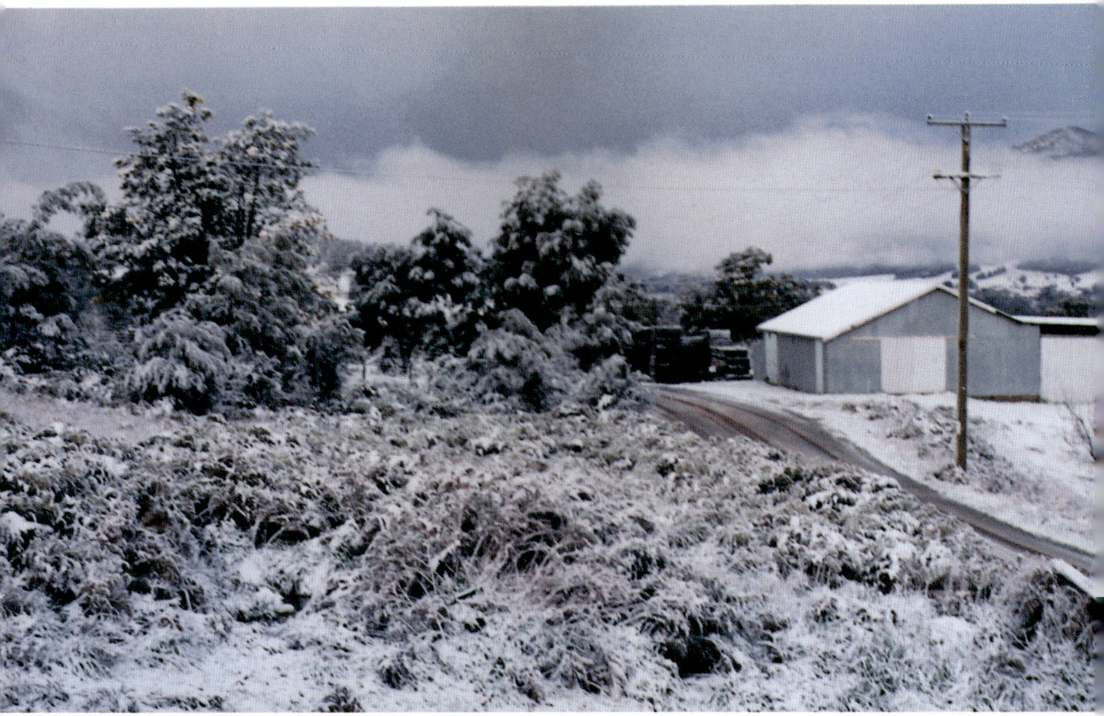

Occasional snowfalls change the Huon into a winter wonderland.

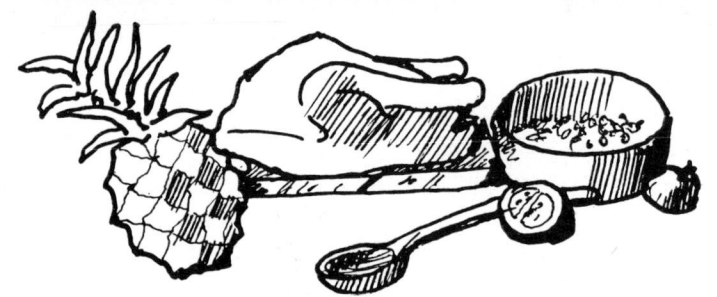

Zucchini Slice

375g zucchini, grated
1 cup cheese, grated
1/2 cup vegetable oil
4 eggs
3 rashers bacon, diced
1 onion, diced
1 cup S.R. flour
Salt & pepper

Mix together zucchini, bacon, cheese, onion & oil; add eggs, then flour, salt & pepper.

Grease casserole dish, pour in mixture; bake in hot oven 30-35 minutes. Can be eaten hot or cold.

Cheesy Egg & Bacon Pie

Cheese Pastry:

1-1/2 cups S.R. flour
1 tablespoon water
Salt
1/3 cup butter
3/4 cup grated cheese

Rub butter into flour with salt; add cheese, mix with water. Knead lightly, roll out, place in 20cm pie plate.

Filling:

6 teaspoons butter
1/2 teaspoon dry mustard
1 dessertspoon chopped parsley
4 rashers bacon, chopped
2 onions, chopped
2-1/2 cups warm milk
3 eggs
Salt & pepper

Fry onions & bacon in butter; add salt, pepper & mustard. Stir well then drain.

Beat eggs in separate bowl, add milk, add parsley, stir in onion & bacon. Place in pastry case; bake in moderate oven 30 to 40 minutes.

Bacon Noodle Patties

1 packet 2 minute noodles
3/4 cup grated potato
4 rashers bacon, chopped
5 eggs, beaten
3 green shallots
60g mushrooms, sliced

Cook noodles then drain. Combine noodles with other ingredients; place 1/4 cup for each pattie in pan then cook in hot oil 3 minutes each side.

Easy Quiche

4 eggs
1 cup bacon, chopped
1/2 cup cheese, grated
1/2 cup S.R. flour
1 cup onion, chopped
1 cup evaporated milk
1 cup fresh milk
Salt & pepper

Mix all ingredients together. Bake in moderate oven until set, about 45 minutes. Serve with salad.

Golden Pumpkin Pie

Pastry:

2-1/2 cups flour
1 tablespoon sugar
4 tablespoons cold water
1/4 teaspoon salt
2/3 cup butter

Mix flour, sugar & salt; rub in butter then mix in water. Knead dough into ball; wrap & chill. When cold roll out thinly; gently ease onto pie plate. Trim and reserve scraps for decorating; chill again. Bake in moderate oven 5 minutes or until golden brown.

Filling:

750g pumpkin, peeled, cubed
1/2 cup golden syrup
1 teaspoon cinnamon
1/2 teaspoon nutmeg
Pinch salt
1 cup milk
2 eggs
3 tablespoons flour
1/2 teaspoon ginger

Steam pumpkin until tender, drain & cool. Mash or blend, beat in milk, eggs & syrup then flour & spices; beat well.

Pour into shell; cook in slow oven 40 to 45 minutes. Pie is cooked when knife inserted into centre comes out clean.

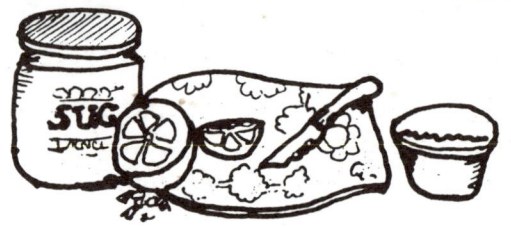

Faye's Fruit Pudding
(Microwave)

Place following ingredients in bowl; microwave on High 3 minutes.

    2 tablespoons butter   1/2 cup brown sugar
    1-1/2 cups mixed fruit   1/4 cup sherry OR brandy OR cold tea

Allow to cool slightly then stir in:

    1 teaspoon bi-carb   1 teaspoon mixed spice
    1 cup S.R. flour   3/4 cup milk

Pour into greased 7 cup pudding bowl; cook uncovered on High 6-1/2 minutes. Cover with upturned plate then cook 1 minute. Allow to cool 1 minute before turning out.

Jelly Slice

Base:
    1 packet milk coffee biscuits   3/4 cup butter, melted

Mix together then press into greased slab tin.

Filling:
    1 tin condensed milk   Juice 2 lemons
    1 dessertspoon gelatine dissolved in 3/4 cup boiling water

Beat together then pour over base. Chill.

Topping:
    Combine 1 packet red jelly & 1-1/2 cups boiling water.

Leave to jell slightly. Pour over filling; leave to set. Cut in squares. Keep in refrigerator.

Blackcurrant Cordial

    2.5kg blackcurrants   18 litres water
    150g citric acid   9kg sugar

Put currants & water in large boiling saucepan, bring to boil; remove from heat, stand overnight. Strain & measure juice, then add citric acid and 500g sugar for each 2-1/2 cups of juice.

Boil 5 minutes. Bottle & seal.

Mrs Lawrence's Pudding

2 cups S.R. flour
3/4 cup warm milk
1/2 teaspoon ginger
2 tablespoons butter
2 tablespoons sugar
1 teaspoon bi-carb
1/2 teaspoon cinnamon
2 tablespoons golden syrup

Place all dry ingredients in bowl. Add butter & golden syrup to warm milk; stir into dry ingredients. Mix well. Place in greased steamer bowl, steam 2 hours.

Baked Apple Roll in Syrup

1 cup flour
1/4 teaspoon soda
Milk
1/2 teaspoon cream of tartar
1/4 cup butter
2 large apples, grated

Mix ingredients together except apple, to form dough. Roll out on floured board. Spread grated apple over, then roll up from long side.

Syrup: 1/2 cup sugar   1 cup hot water
6 teaspoons butter

Mix all together, pour over roll in ovenproof dish. Bake in slow oven 45 minutes.

Baked Fudge Pudding

1 cup S.R. flour
2 tablespoons cocoa
2 tablespoons melted butter
3/4 cup sugar
1/2 cup milk

Mix all together, place in ovenproof dish.
Topping: 3/4 cup brown sugar   1/4 cup cocoa
1-1/4 cups boiling water

Mix together, pour over base mixture. Bake in moderate oven 35 minutes.

Country Apple Crumble

Peel & slice 6 large apples; cook in a little water until soft; place in pie dish, sprinkle cinnamon.
Topping: 1-1/2 cups S.R. flour   1/2 cup coconut
3/4 cup brown sugar   1/3 cup butter

Mix all ingredients together; sprinkle over apple. Bake in moderate oven 20 minutes.

Steamed Choc Pudding

1/2 cup sugar
1-1/2 cups flour
1/2 teaspoon cream of tartar
1 tablespoon cocoa
2 tablespoons milk

1/2 teaspoon soda
1/2 cup butter, melted
2 eggs
Vanilla

Beat together eggs, sugar, milk & butter. Mix in dry ingredients, beat well. Place in steamer, cover; steam 1-1/2 hours. Serve with lots of cream.

Mum's Meringue

3 egg whites
1 teaspoon vinegar
Pinch salt

3/4 cup castor sugar
1 teaspoon vanilla

Beat egg whites with salt until stiff; add sugar then beat again; trickle in vinegar & vanilla while beating. Place on tray, spread into even layer; bake in very cool oven 2-1/2 hours.

Nan Rob's Boston Pudding

1-1/2 cups flour
1 tablespoon raspberry jam
1/2 cup butter/margarine
1 teaspoon cinnamon
1 cup cold tea

1 cup mixed fruit
1/2 cup sugar
1 teaspoon soda
1/2 teaspoon nutmeg

Melt butter, add sugar, jam, cold tea, & fruit. Stir in dry ingredients, mix well. Place in large greased steamer bowl, steam 1-1/2 hours. Serve with custard.

Pineapple Fluff

1 small can pineapple, diced
3/4 cup sugar
1/2 dessertspoon gelatine

3/4 cup hot water
2 eggs

Dissolve gelatine in hot water. Beat egg whites & sugar until stiff; beat yolks separately. Drain pineapple, add to yolks, mix in gelatine quickly, fold in egg whites. Chill.

Golden Pudding

1 cup S.R. flour
1/2 cup sugar
2 tablespoons golden syrup
1/2 cup milk
1 egg
1/4 cup butter

Beat butter with sugar & egg, add milk then lastly flour. Beat well. Cover bottom of greased basin with golden syrup then pour mixture over. Steam 1 hour. Serve with custard.

Ice Cream Whip

1 cup evaporated milk, chilled
1 tablespoon gelatine
Vanilla
1/2 cup sugar
3/4 cup hot water

Dissolve gelatine in water. Beat milk until thick, add sugar then beat again; dribble in vanilla & gelatine mix while still beating. Place in serving bowl, chill. Can be flavoured if wished, e.g. cocoa, raspberries, peppermint.

Date Sponge Pudding

1 cup S.R. flour
1/2 cup sugar
2 tablespoons milk
Vanilla essence
1 egg
2 teaspoons butter
1/2 cup dates, chopped

Beat together sugar, butter & egg, add milk, vanilla, dates; stir in flour, mix well. Put into steamer, cover; steam 1 hour. Serve with custard.

Boiled Apple Pudding

Peel, core & slice apples. Put in saucepan with little water & sugar. Make topping:

1/2 cup S.R. flour
1 tablespoon sugar
1 egg, well beaten

Mix all ingredients together then put mixture over apples. Steam & juice from apple will cook topping. Add little milk only if necessary; mix should not be too moist. Cover and boil slowly 30 minutes.

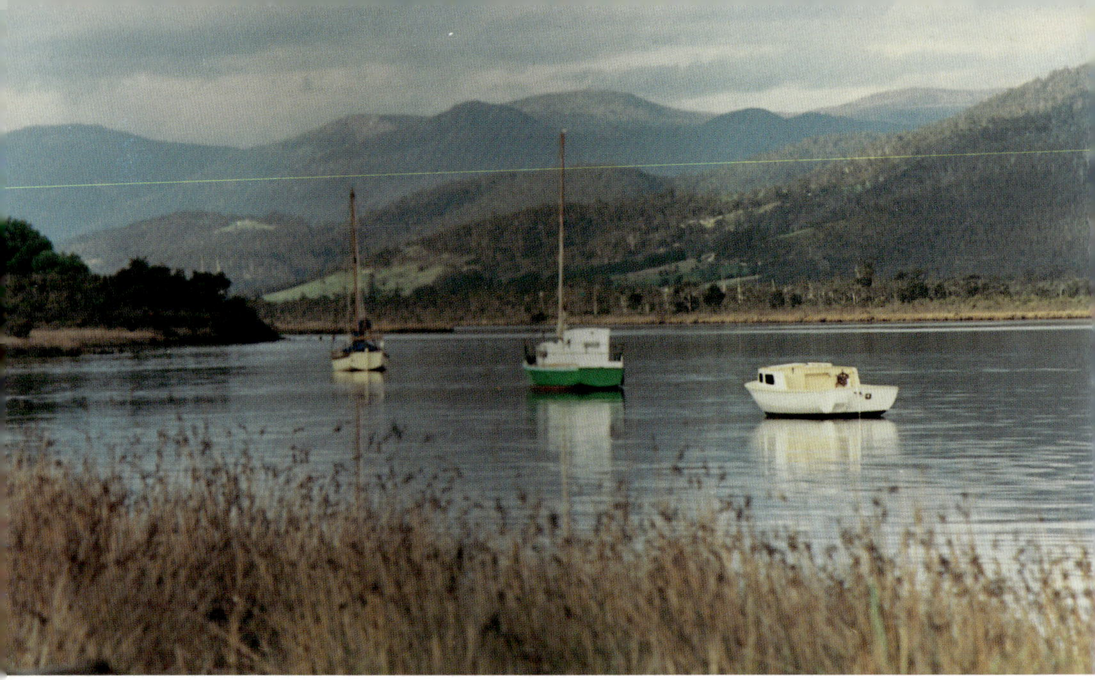

The Huon River once was the only means of access to the valley, it is still important for its fish farms and deep sea ports.

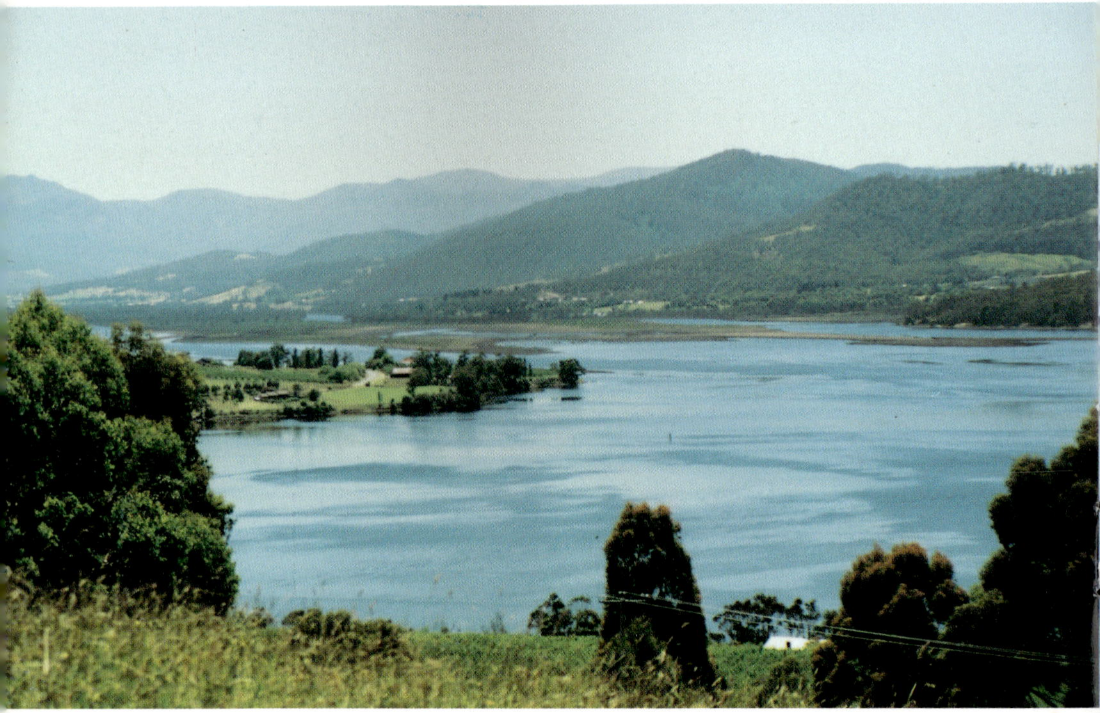

Originally tall timber grew to the river edge. Egg Island provides an extensive wildlife refuge; distinctive black swans abound.

No Bake Lemon Velvet Pie

Crust: 1 packet milk coffee biscuits   1/2 cup butter
1/2 teaspoon nutmeg

Crush biscuits, add melted butter & nutmeg. Press mixture firmly into greased pie plate, then chill.

Filling: 1 teaspoon gelatine   2 tablespoons hot water
3/4 cup lemon spread   1 cup cream

Dissolve gelatine in water. Add to lemon spread; stir until smooth. Whip cream, fold into lemon mix; pour into pie crust. Chill before serving. Best if made the day before using.

Apple Meringue Pie

1/2 packet coffee biscuits   1/4 cup butter, melted
6 teaspoons sugar

Crush biscuits, mix with sugar & butter. Press into 20cm pie dish; bake in moderate oven 10 minutes. Allow to cool.

Filling: 3 large apples, stewed   1 egg yolk
1/3 cup sugar   6 teaspoons cornflour

To warm apple add egg yolk, sugar & cornflour; mix well. Place on stove, cook 5 minutes, stirring continually. Allow to cool.

Topping: 1 egg white   1/4 cup sugar

Beat egg white & sugar until soft peaks form. Pour filling into pie shell, top with meringue. Bake in slow oven 20 to 30 minutes or until golden brown. Serve cold.

Jam Roll

2 cups S.R. flour   Pinch salt
1/2 cup butter   1 cup milk or water

Rub butter into flour with salt until it resembles breadcrumbs, mix in enough milk to make soft dough; roll out on floured board. Cut into three pieces, spread each with different jam (e.g. raspberry, blackberry, apricot).

Fold sides to centre and fold ends in to retain jam. Place on tray then bake in very hot oven 10 to 15 minutes. Serve with custard.

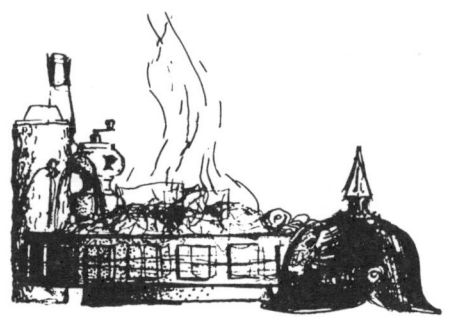

Quick Steamed Pudding (1)

Beat together: 1 egg & 1/4 cup sugar
Add: 1/4 cup milk & 1/2 cup S.R. flour, alternately
Dissolve: 1 teaspoon butter in 1 teaspoon boiling water, then add to mixture

Beat well. Place raspberry jam in bottom of steamer; top with mixture; steam 30 minutes.

Quick Steamed Pudding (2)

1 cup S.R. flour	1 dessertspoon sugar
1 dessertspoon butter	1 egg
1 cup milk	Pinch salt

Place flour & sugar in basin, rub in butter, add salt. Beat egg in cup and fill cup with milk; mix all together.
Place jam or golden syrup in bottom of steamer, pour mixture over and boil 30 minutes.

Apricot Mousse

Microwave

825g tinned apricots	2 teaspoons gelatine
300g carton sour cream	

Drain apricots, reserve syrup. Over 1/2 cup syrup sprinkle gelatine; microwave on High 1 minute, cool to room temperature.
Puree apricots in blender, add sour cream & gelatine mixture; blend until smooth. Pour into serving dishes, chill until set. Decorate with sliced apricots & whipped cream.

Bread & Butter Custard

8 eggs
1 teaspoon vanilla
1/2 cup sultanas
1/2 cup coconut, grated
Sliced bread

1 cup sugar
1 litre milk
Little butter
Sprinkle nutmeg

Beat eggs with sugar & vanilla; slowly add milk. Pour into 2 litre casserole dish; add sultanas. Butter enough slices of bread to cover dish, cut into 1/4's and place on top of custard. Cover thickly with coconut, sprinkle nutmeg.

Place in pan of water, cook in moderate oven 45 minutes or until golden brown. Custard is cooked when knife stuck into centre comes out clean.

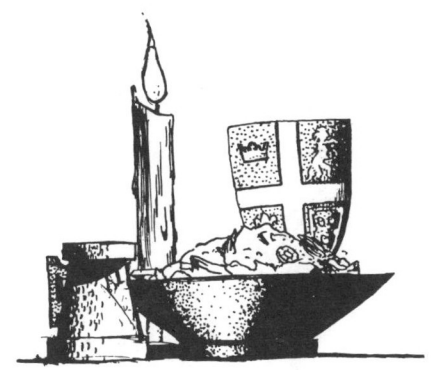

Quick Christmas Pudding

Boil together:
    2 cups milk   1/2 cup butter   2 teaspoons bi-carb

Add:
    2 cups S.R. flour   1 teaspoon cinnamon
    1 cup brown sugar   1 tablespoon mixed spice
    1/2 packet raisins   1 packet mixed fruit
    1/2 teaspoon vanilla & almond essence

Mix well then turn into greased pudding basin; cover. Boil 2-1/2 to 3 hours. Re boil 1/2 to 3/4 hour before serving.

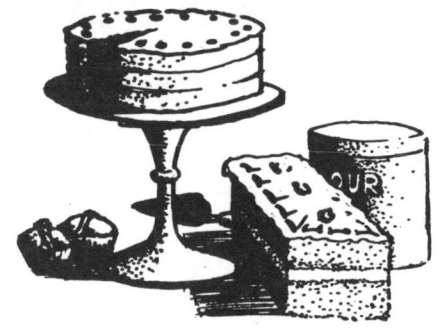

Raspberry Shortcake

2 eggs
1/2 cup butter
1 cup coconut
1-3/4 cups sugar
1-1/2 cups S.R. flour

Rub butter into flour & 3/4 cup sugar, mix in 1 egg. Roll out, press in rectangular tin, then spread with raspberry jam. Mix together 1 cup sugar, coconut & 1 egg; spread on top of jam. Bake in slow oven 3/4 hour.

Apple Shortcake

2 cups S.R. flour
1 cup sugar
1/2 cup butter
Cinnamon to sprinkle
1 egg
Milk to bind
2 cups stewed apple

Rub butter into flour & sugar; add egg & milk. Line tin with half of mixture; cover with stewed apple, then rest of mixture. Bake in moderate oven 20 to 30 minutes. Ice then sprinkle cinnamon.
Icing: Beat together: 1 cup icing sugar
 1 dessertspoon butter
 Juice 1 lemon OR 1/2 teaspoon vanilla with little milk

Tea Cake

1/2 cup sugar
1/2 cup milk
1-1/2 cups S.R. flour
1 egg
2 dessertspoons butter

Cream butter & sugar, add egg, milk, & flour last. Place in greased 20cm round cake tin then sprinkle with sugar & cinnamon. Bake in moderate oven 25 minutes.

Connie's Sponge Cake

4 eggs
2 teaspoons glycerine
1 cup cornflour
1/2 teaspoon bi-carb
Vanilla
3/4 cup sugar
1 teaspoon cream of tartar

Sift dry ingredients together three times. Separate eggs then beat whites until stiff. Beat egg yolks & sugar; add dry ingredients, fold in glycerine; lastly fold in egg whites.

Place in greased, floured 20cm baking tin then bake in moderate oven 15 minutes or until cake leaves sides of tin.

Blackberry & Apple Sponge

6 large apples, stewed
1 egg
1 cup S.R. flour
Vanilla
2 cups blackberries
1/2 cup sugar
1/2 to 1 cup milk
Icing sugar to sprinkle

Place alternate layers of apple & blackberries in pie dish. Beat egg, sugar & vanilla, add flour & milk alternately, keeping mix to pouring consistency. Pour over fruit then bake in hot oven 20 to 25 minutes.

Sprinkle icing sugar.

Sponge Cake

3 eggs
1 cup flour
1 teaspoon baking powder
1 dessertspoon butter
1 cup sugar
2 teaspoons cornflour
6 tablespoons milk

Put butter & milk on to boil. Separate eggs; beat whites until stiff, add sugar then beat again. Add yolks & vanilla then fold in flour; add boiling milk & butter.

Place in greased & floured 20cm tins, bake in hot oven 10 minutes.

Basic Butter Icing:

1 tablespoon butter
1 tablspoon milk
1 cup icing sugar
1/4 teaspoon vanilla

Cream butter until white & smooth. Add vanilla & icing sugar; add milk only necessary to make spreading consistency. Can be flavoured as desired.

York Cherry Cake

1 cup butter
4 eggs
1/3 cup cherries
1 cup sugar
2-1/2 cups flour
1 teaspoon baking powder

Cream butter & sugar, add beaten eggs & flour, cherries & baking powder. Mix well. Turn into greased & paper lined 20cm baking tin. Bake in moderate oven 1-1/2 hours.

Lemon Shortbread

1/2 cup butter
1/2 cup sugar
1 egg
2 cups S.R. flour

Cream butter & sugar, add egg, mix in flour. Roll out then cut in bars to size required. Cook in moderate oven 20 minutes.

Icing: Juice of 1 lemon 1 teaspoon butter
3/4 cup icing sugar

Mix together and use to join biscuits or ice tops.

Jill's Cheesecake

Crust: 1 pkt coffee biscuits, crushed 1/2 cup brown sugar
2 teaspoons ginger 3/4 cup melted butter
Mix all together, place in spring form tin then chill.

Filling: 1/2 cup water 3 teaspoons gelatine
1/2 cup evaporated milk

Heat water in saucepan, dissolve gelatine. Take off heat; add milk; put aside to begin to thicken.

Add: 1/2 cup chilled evaporated milk 1/2 cup sugar
250g Philadelphia cheese 1/4 cup dry cocoa
4 drops peppermint essence Green food colouring
1/4 teaspoon vanilla

Beat cheese with sugar & vanilla, beat milk until thick then mix with cheese; add gelatine mix.

Divide mixture equally in two bowls. To one add cocoa; beat well. To other add peppermint & green colour. Spoon mixtures alternately into crust to give marble effect. Place in refrigerator to set. Decorate with whipped cream & finely chopped peppermint crisps.

Chocolate Apple Cake

1 cup sugar	1/2 cup margarine
2 cups S.R. flour	1-1/2 cups stewed apple
250g sultanas	1/2 teaspoon cinnamon
5 teaspoons cocoa	2 teaspoons soda

Add soda to warm apple. Cream butter & sugar; add apple, fruit & dry ingredients.

Place in greased, lined square tin then bake in moderate oven 30-45 minutes.

Chocolate Walnut Cake

1 large cup flour	1 cup sugar
2 eggs	1 cup butter
1/2 teaspoon bi-carb	1 tablespoon cocoa
1/2 cup warm milk	1 tablespoon golden syrup
Vanilla	1/2 cup chopped walnuts

Cream butter & sugar; add eggs then nuts, golden syrup, cocoa, flour; lastly dissolve bi-carb in milk. Mix well. Put in greased, floured 20cm deep round cake tin. Cook in moderate oven 1 hour.

Ice with chocolate icing, sprinkle walnuts.

Rich Chocolate Cake

(Makes 2)

2-1/4 cups S.R. flour	2/3 cup butter
1-3/4 cups sugar	1 cup water
1 teaspoon bi-carb	1 teaspoon vanilla
2/3 cup cocoa	3 eggs

Soften butter; place all ingredients except eggs into bowl. Beat 3 minutes, add eggs 1 at a time, continue to beat for further 3 minutes.

Pour into 2 well greased 20cm cake tins; bake in moderate oven 35 to 40 minutes. When cold slice each cake then fill with whipped cream; ice with rich choc icing. Can be filled, iced and frozen.

Coconut Cake
(Slab tin)

2 cups flour
1 cup sugar
2 tablespoons coconut
2 teaspoons baking powder

1/2 cup butter
3/4 cup milk
2 eggs

Melt butter then mix in all other ingredients. Bake in moderate oven 20 minutes. Ice with vanilla icing; top with coconut.

Icing: Beat together: 1 tablespoon butter   1 teaspoon vanilla
1 cup icing sugar   Little milk

Coconut Ice Cake

125g butter
1-1/2 cups flour
2 eggs

2/3 cup sugar
3 teaspoons milk
2 tablespoons coconut

Soften butter then mix all ingredients together. Colour half mixture pink then place in alternate layers in cake tin. Bake in moderate oven 35 minutes.

Butterscotch Cake

1 cup brown sugar
1 teaspoon vanilla
2 eggs, separated
1/2 cup milk

1/2 cup butter
1-1/4 cups S.R. flour
1 tablespoon golden syrup
1/2 teaspoon cinnamon

Cream butter & sugar; add yolks then beat well. Stir in syrup, milk & vanilla; add dry ingredients. Beat egg whites stiff; fold into mixture. Pour into 18cm, deep square cake tin. Bake in moderate oven 20 to 30 minutes.

Ice when not quite cold.

Icing: 1 cup brown sugar   3 tablespoons milk
1 teaspoon butter   1/4 teaspoon vanilla

Boil together 5 minutes; beat until thick then spread over warm cake.

Orange Cake

1/3 cup melted butter
3/4 cup sugar
1-1/2 cups S.R. flour
4 tablespoons milk
Juice & rind 1 orange
2 eggs

Mix all ingredients together 3 minutes.
Bake in moderate oven 30 minutes.
Ice with orange icing & sprinkle grated rind.

Icing: Blend together:
1 tablespoon butter
1 cup icing sugar
Juice 1/2 orange

Raspberry Cake

1/2 cup butter
1/2 cup sugar
1 egg
1 cup icing sugar
1 cup S.R. flour
3 tablespoons milk
Raspberry jam

Cream butter & sugar, add egg & milk then flour. Beat well. Place half mixture in 20cm round cake tin, spread with raspberry jam then place rest of mixture on top. Bake in moderate oven 30 minutes.

When cold, ice with 1 cup icing sugar mixed with 1 tablespoon raspberry jam & little butter.

Marshmallow Cake

3 weetbix
1 cup S.R. flour
3/4 cup brown sugar
1/2 cup butter, melted
1 cup coconut
1/2 teaspoon vanilla

Crush weetbix, mix all ingredients together. Press into shallow tin then bake in slow oven 1/2 hour. Cool in tin.
Boil together: 3/4 cup sugar   1 cup water
   1 tablespoon gelatine
Cook 5 minutes, allow to cool slightly, beat until thick; colour if desired. Pour into crust; sprinkle coconut or 100's & 1000's; cut into slices.

Light Fruit Cake

3/4 cup butter
3 eggs
1 cup plain flour
Little milk

3/4 cup sugar
1 cup S.R.flour
2-2/3 cups mixed fruit
Vanilla

Soften butter then mix all ingredients together, adding fruit last, DO NOT OVER MIX. Bake in moderate oven 1 hour 15 minutes. Cool in tin 10 minutes before turning out.

One-Two-Three-Four Cake

1 cup butter   2 cups sugar   3 cups flour   4 eggs
2 teaspoons baking powder   Pinch salt
Little milk
1-1/2 cups mixed fruit OR 1-1/2 cups coconut OR rind & juice 1 orange OR 2 tablespoons caraway seeds

Cream butter & sugar, add all other ingredients. Place in greased, floured 20cm deep cake tin, bake in moderate oven 45 minutes.

Caraway Seed Cake

1/2 cup milk
1 cup sugar
2 eggs
1/2 cup butter

1-1/3 cups S.R. flour
2 tablespoons custard powder
2 tablespoons caraway seeds

Beat butter, sugar, eggs & milk; add flour & custard powder. Beat 3 minutes then stir in seeds. Grease large square tin, cover base with greased paper. Pour in mixture then bake in slow oven 1 hour. Let stand 5 minutes before turning out to cool.

Buried Dates

1-1/2 cups S.R. flour
125g butter
Vanilla

1/2 cup sugar
1 egg
Dates, stoned

Rub butter into flour & sugar, add egg & vanilla. Roll each date in piece of dough, roll in sugar then place on greased tray. Bake in hot oven 10 minutes.

Rock Cakes

125g butter
2 cups S.R. flour
1 teaspoon vanilla
Pinch salt

1-1/2 cups mixed fruit
1/2 cup sugar
2 eggs

Cream butter & sugar, add eggs, flour & fruit. Drop teaspoonsful on greased tray, bake in moderate oven 10-15 minutes or until brown.

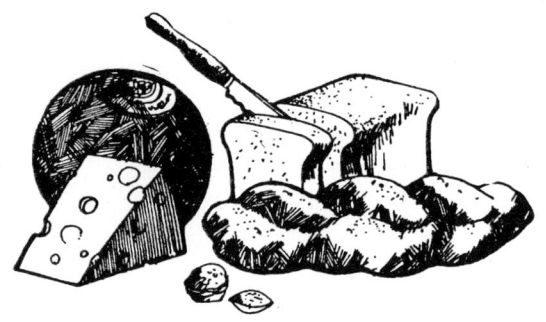

Scone Savoury

1 cup milk
1 cup S.R. flour
1 cup cheese, grated

1/2 onion, grated
1 rasher bacon, chopped
1 teaspoon parsley

Mix all ingredients together; place in greased gem irons or shallow patty tins.
Cook in hot oven 7 to 10 minutes. When cold, split then spread with butter.

Pumpkin Scones

2 cups S.R. flour
1/2 cup sugar
1 cup cooked mashed pumpkin

Pinch salt
1 egg
1 tablespoon butter

Beat butter and sugar to cream. Add egg, beat well; add pumpkin then fold in flour & salt. Turn onto floured board, pat or roll to 1cm thick. Cut in shapes with knife or floured scone cutter, then place on lightly greased tray. Cook in hot oven 10 minutes.

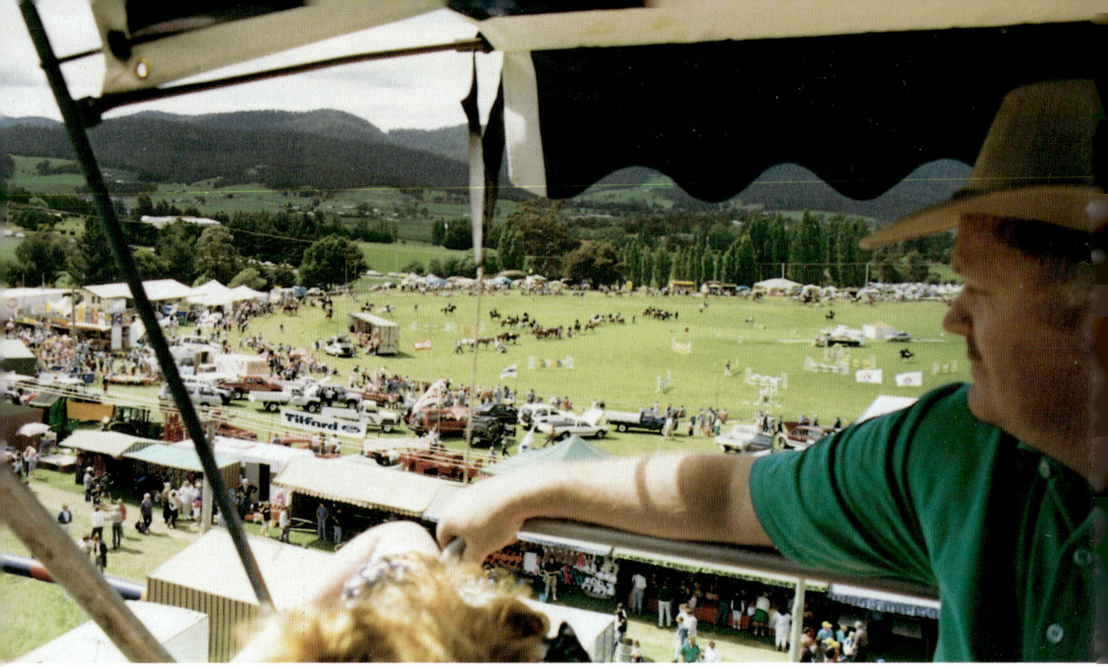

The annual Huon Show features all the traditional attractions.

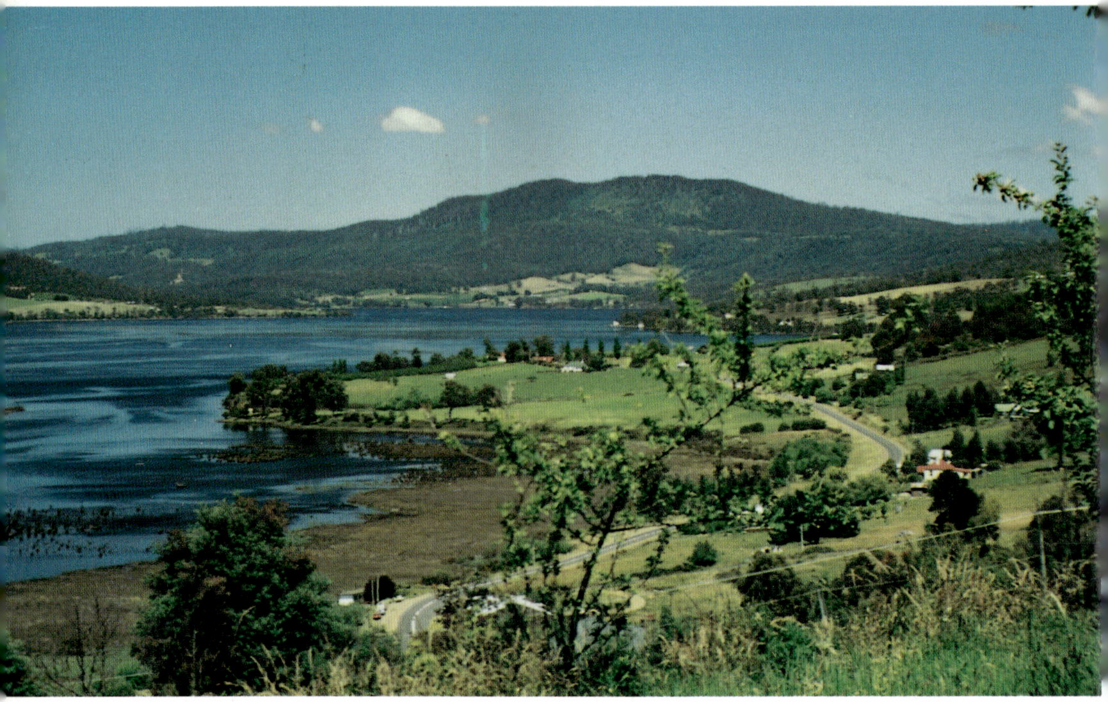

Castle Forbes Bay, named after an immigrant sailing ship which came up the river in error, mistaking it for the Derwent River.

Sultana Scones

3 cups S.R. flour
1/2 teaspoon salt
1/4 cup butter
1/4 cup sugar
1 cup sultanas
1 egg, beaten
1 cup milk

Rub butter into flour & salt, add sugar & sultanas. Make well in centre, add egg & enough milk to make soft dough. Roll out 2cm thick on floured board; cut into rounds. Bake in very hot oven 15 minutes.

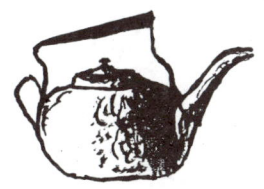

Zucchini Bread

3 eggs
2 teaspoons vanilla
1 teaspoon salt
1 teaspoon bi-carb
3 teaspoons cinnamon
1 cup chopped walnuts
1-1/2 cups raw sugar
1 cup margarine or peanut oil
2 large cups zucchini, grated
3 cups wholemeal flour
1/4 teaspoon baking powder

Grease 2 cake tins. Beat eggs and sugar, add vanilla & oil, beat again. Stir in zucchini, fold in flour & nuts. Bake in moderate oven 1 to 1-1/2 hours. Slice and butter when cold.

Gingerbread Loaf

2-1/4 cups flour
1 teaspoon bi-carb
1 teaspoon nutmeg
3 teaspoons ginger
1/2 teaspoon salt
1 egg, beaten

Melt together: 1/2 cup butter
2 tablespoons golden syrup
1 cup brown sugar
1/2 cup water

When cool add egg & dry ingredients; mix well. Place in greased, floured loaf tin, bake in moderate oven 1-1/2 hours.

Brown Loaf

1-1/2 cups water
1-1/4 cups sugar
1-1/4 cups mixed fruit
2 tablespoons butter
2 tablespoons mixed peel

Put all ingredients in saucepan then boil 5 minutes. When cold add:

2-3/4 cups flour
1/2 teaspoon cinnamon
1 teaspoon bi-carb
1 teaspoon spice

Place in greased, floured loaf tin, bake in moderate oven 45 minutes. Keeps well.

Date Loaf

1 cup dates
1 teaspoon mixed spice
3 tablespoons butter
2-1/2 cups S.R. flour
1 teaspoon bi-carb
1 cup boiling water
1 cup sugar

Boil all ingredients together exept flour. Let cool then add flour; place in greased, floured loaf tin then bake in moderate oven 1 hour.

Raisin or Nut Loaf

1 cup water
1 cup dates, raisins OR nuts
1 teaspoon bi-carb
Pinch salt
2 cups S.R. flour
1 cup sugar
1 tablespoon butter
1 egg, beaten

Put water, sugar, fruit, soda & butter on to boil 1 minute. Remove from heat to add flour, salt & egg. Place in greased, floured loaf tin; bake in moderate oven 45 minutes.

Quick Choc Loaf

1 cup S.R. flour
1/4 cup cocoa
1 cup sugar
1/2 cup milk
1/2 teaspoon vanilla
2 eggs
1/2 cup butter, softened

Place all ingredients in bowl; beat well then pour into greased loaf tin. Bake in moderate oven 35-40 minutes.

Poor Man's Loaf

1 cup hot tea
1 cup sultanas
1 cup sugar
1 cup S.R. flour
1 cup plain flour

Soak sugar & sultanas in tea until cool (not cold). Mix in flours. Place in greased loaf pan; bake in hot oven 45 minutes or until golden brown. Loaf will rise then split in middle (this is normal); it will leave sides of tin when cooked.

Slice, spread with butter; use hot or cold.

Four In One Biscuits

250g S.R. flour
125g butter
125g sugar

Vanilla
1 egg
1/4 cup milk

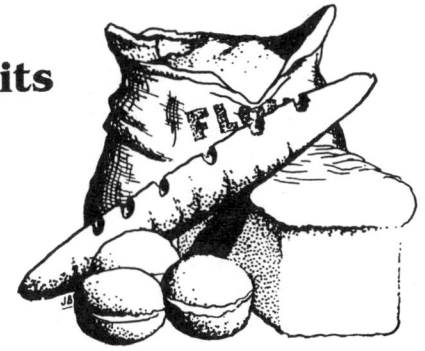

Cream butter & sugar, add egg & vanilla. Then add flour & milk alternately. Drop teaspoonsful on greased tray, bake in moderate oven 10 minutes.

Currant Spice : add 1 cup currants, 2 teaspoons cinnamon
Fruit Cookies: add 1 cup mixed fruit
Choc Cookies: add 1/4 cup cocoa

Coconut Jam Drops

1/2 cup margarine
3/4 cup sugar
1 teaspoon cream of tartar
1/2 teaspoon bi-carb
2 eggs
2 tablespoons coconut
2 cups flour

Cream butter & sugar, add eggs & dry ingredients. Form into balls, press dent in centre. Fill dent with jam, pinch together then roll in sugar. Bake in medium oven 15 minutes.

Alana's Monte Carlos

1/2 cup butter
1 egg
1-1/2 cups S.R. flour
1/4 cup sugar
3 teaspoons honey
3 teaspoons custard powder

Cream butter with sugar; mix with other ingredients. Roll into balls, place on tray, press down with fork. Bake in moderate oven 10 minutes or until golden brown. Join together with vanilla icing & raspberry jam.

Icing: Beat together: 1 tablespoon butter   Little milk
1 teaspoon vanilla   1 cup icing sugar

Choc-Chip Biscuits

2/3 cup butter
1/2 cup sugar
2 cups S.R. flour
1 packet choc bits
2 eggs

Melt butter in saucepan, add sugar then stir until dissolved; allow to cool. Beat in eggs, flour & choc bits. Drop teaspoonsful on greased tray. Bake in moderate oven 15 minutes. Cool before removing from tray.

Milo Biscuits

1/2 cup butter
2 tablespoons Milo
1 cup coconut
2 cups S.R. flour
1/2 cup sugar

Cream butter & sugar, add egg; stir in flour, milo, & coconut. Put teaspoonsful on greased tray. Bake in moderate oven 15 to 20 minutes; will burn quickly once cooked - watch carefully.

Kiss Biscuits

Beat 1 cup butter & 1 cup sugar to a cream; add 3 eggs (1 at a time). Beat well, then add 3 cups flour with 2 teaspoons cream of tartar & 1 teaspoon bi-carb added. Blend well. Roll out, cut into rounds then bake in moderate oven until golden brown.

When cold fill with raspberry jam, ice with vanilla icing; top with 100's & 1000's or coconut.

Ginger Creams

2-1/2 cups flour
1 cup sugar
1 cup butter
1 teaspoon bi-carb
1 tablespoon golden syrup
1 egg
1-1/2 teaspoons ground ginger

Cream butter & sugar, add egg & golden syrup, then dry ingredients. Put teaspoonsful on lightly greased oven slide then bake in moderate oven 10 to 15 minutes or until golden.

Join together with butter icing.

Icing: Mix together: 3/4 cup icing sugar   Little milk
1 tablespoon butter

Butter-Nut Biscuits

2 tablespoons butter
1 cup sugar
1 egg
1/2 teaspoon vanilla
2 tablespoons golden syrup
1-1/2 tablespoons milk
1-1/2 cups S.R. flour
1 cup coconut
Pinch salt

Cream butter & sugar with vanilla, add golden syrup, then egg & milk; fold in dry ingredients. Roll into balls, place on tray then press with fork. Bake in moderate oven 15 to 20 minutes.

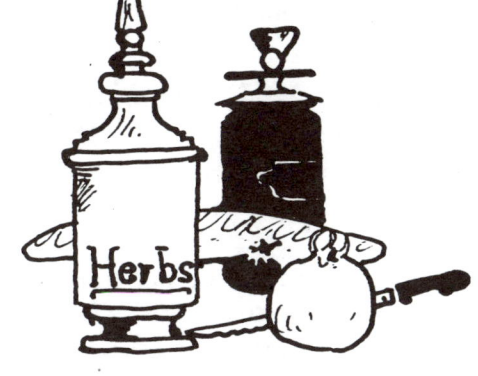

Apple Jam

6 apples, chopped   2 lemons, sliced
1-1/2 cups sugar to each 500g fruit

Cover chopped apple with water; boil 45 minutes. Add sugar, then lemon. Boil gently 2 hours. Bottle & seal.

Raspberry Jam

1kg raspberries 1kg sugar, warm
Juice 1 lemon

Heat fruit gently in saucepan until juice begins to run. Add sugar slowly, stirring until dissolved. Add lemon juice; boil until setting. Bottle in airtight container.

Apple Jelly

Small green apples Sugar
Water

Core, quarter apples, cover with water. Simmer 30 minutes, strain off liquid through fine strainer; add 2 cups sugar to each 2-1/2 cups liquid. Boil 20 to 30 minutes or until it jells. Bottle & seal.

Melon & Lemon Jam

To every 2.5kg melon, cut in pieces, allow 2.5kg sugar & 3 lemons, sliced.
Put half sugar over melon, leave overnight. In separate dish put lemon & 3 cups boiling water, leave overnight.
Mix all together, bring to boil, add remaining sugar, boil until clear amber colour. Bottle & seal.

Lemon Butter

3 lemons, washed 2/3 cup butter
3 eggs 500g castor sugar
Grated rind of half lemons

Put sugar, juice of lemons & grated rind in top of double boiler. Place over gently boiling water; stir until sugar dissolved. Remove from heat, allow to cool.
Whisk eggs thoroughly, then strain into lemon mixture; stir thoroughly. Return to boiling water to simmer while stirring, about 15 minutes or until mixture is thick as honey. Cool slightly before storing in clean, dry jars, in cool place or refrigerator.

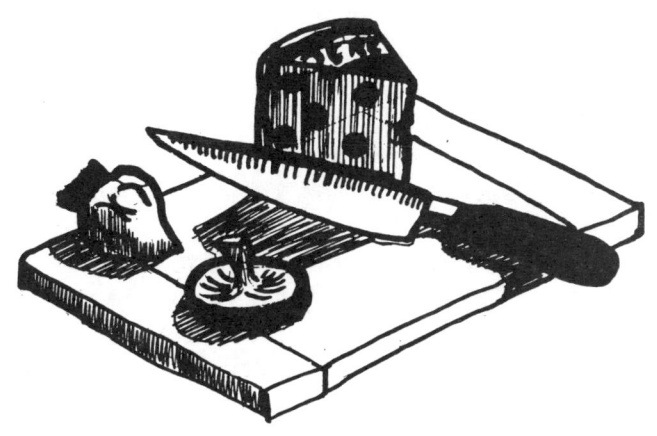

Cheese Sauce

1 cup grated cheddar cheese
1 teaspoon lemon rind
1-1/2 cups milk
1 tablespoon cornflour

Blend cornflour & milk together until smooth; bring to boil, stirring constantly. Add lemon rind & cheese; lower heat, then stir until cheese melts.

Chocolate Sauce

1 tablespoon cocoa
1 cup hot water
1 tablespoon golden syrup
1 tablespoon butter
1 cup sugar
Vanilla essence

Combine butter, cocoa & water; bring to boil, add sugar & golden syrup; boil 5 minutes without stirring, then add vanilla.

Caramel Sauce

30g butter or margarine
Small tin reduced cream
1 cup brown sugar

Melt butter or margarine in saucepan; add sugar. Stir over low heat until sugar dissolves, then add reduced cream all at once. Remove from heat and stir until cream dissolves and sauce thickens slightly.

Plum Sauce

1.5kg plums
2 cups sugar
2 teaspoons green ginger
12 whole cloves

2 cups white vinegar
1 teaspoon salt
1/2 teaspoon cinnamon
1/2 teaspoon pepper

Put plums, vinegar, sugar, salt, cinnamon & pepper in large boiler. Tie cloves & ginger loosly in muslin bag, add to pan. Bring to boil, reduce heat, simmer gently without lid 2 hours. Strain to remove skins & seeds.
Bottle in sterilised jars; seal.

Cabbage & Mustard Pickle

1 large cabbage
1 cup salt
1 cup flour
1 teaspoon curry powder
4 large onions

1 litre vinegar
2 cups sugar
2 teaspoons mustard
600ml vinegar (to mix)

Cut cabbage finely with onions, sprinkle salt, allow to stand 24 hours. Drain well then boil in 1 litre vinegar for 20 minutes. Mix flour, sugar, curry & mustard with remaining vinegar. Add to cabbage then boil 5 minutes.
Place in sterilised jars, seal tightly.

Cauliflower Pickle

1 large cauliflower
9 cups vinegar
2 tablespoons mustard
3/4 cup plain flour

2 cups salt
500g onions, chopped
1 tablespoon tumeric
4 cups sugar

Break cauliflower into sections; place in saucepan of boiling water to which salt has been added. Boil 1 minute, then strain.
Boil vinegar with onions. Blend mustard, tumeric, flour & sugar together with 1 cup vinegar until smooth, then add to boiling vinegar & onions. Boil 2 minutes; add drained cauliflower, bring back to boil. Remove from heat, bottle in sterilised jars; seal.

Fruit Chocs

100g dark chocolate
*Dried apricot, chopped
*Crushed nuts

2 cups sultanas
*Coconut

Melt chocolate; have ready in bowl sultanas & other dried fruits (*these can be varied to suit taste). Pour chocolate over, mix quickly, place in paper cases. Set at room temperature. Can be frozen.

Snowballs

1/4 cup butter
1 egg
1 cup flour

1/4 cup sugar
3 tablespoons milk
1 teaspoon vanilla

Cream butter & sugar & vanilla, add egg then beat well. Add flour & milk alternately. Grease shallow patty tins then place 1 teaspoon of mix in each. Bake 8 to 10 minutes in very hot oven. Ice & roll in coconut. Can be rolled in jelly & coconut, split then filled with cream.

Coconut Rough

1/2 cup coconut to each 100g milk chocolate

Place coconut on small flat dish; toast under grill or in oven (once dried it will burn quickly).

Melt chocolate; combine with coconut. Place teaspoonsful on metal tray which has been chilled beforehand; leave to set.

Rocky Road

1 packet pink marshmallow
1 cup rice bubbles
1/2 cup coconut

1/2 cup peanuts (optional)
200g chocolate (dark or milk)

Melt chocolate. Mix all other ingredients together; mix with chocolate. Press into greased tray, allow to set. Cut into slices.

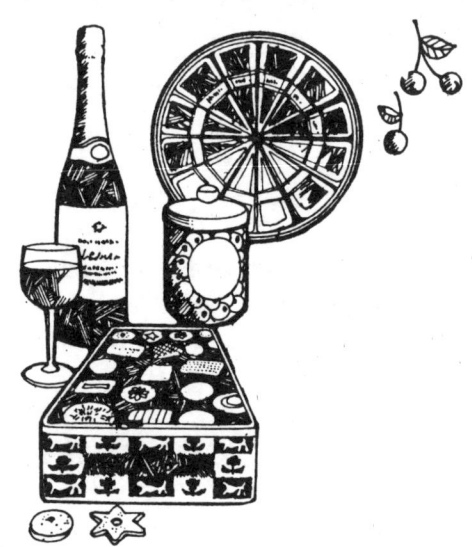

Gingerbread Men

1 egg
1 cup sugar
1 teaspoon salt
1 teaspoon baking powder
1/2 teaspoon ground ginger
1 tablespoon lemon rind & juice

30g butter
1/2 cup honey
3 cups flour
1/2 teaspoon cinnamon
3/4 teaspoon nutmeg

Combine sugar, honey, butter & lemon in saucepan over low heat. Allow to cool, add egg.

Sift other ingredients into bowl, then add mixture from saucepan. Knead into soft dough, chill 30 minutes, then roll out on floured board; cut out shapes. Bake in moderately slow oven 15 minutes. Decorate with smarties etc.

Caramels

1/2 cup butter
1-1/2 cups brown sugar

1 tin condensed milk
Vanilla essence

Melt butter in saucepan, add condensed milk; mix well. Add few drops vanilla & sugar, stirring with wooden spoon until melted. Bring to boil, cook quickly 5 minutes, stirring often. Pour into well greased shallow tin; cut into squares with sharp knife just before it sets.

Some Quick Cup Measures
1 cup of:

flour	150g	fresh breadcrumbs	60g
white sugar	210g	dry breadcrumbs	125g
icing sugar	150g	biscuit crumbs	105g
brown sugar	150g	rice, raw	180g
butter	210g	mixed fruit	185g
honey	360g	nuts, chopped	125g
coconut, dried	90g	cheddar cheese, grated	150g

Measures

LIQUID		SOLID	
Imperial	Metric	Ounces	Grams
1 teaspoon	5ml	1oz	30g
1 tablespoon	20ml	4oz (1/4lb)	125g
2 fluid oz (1/4 cup)	62.5ml	8oz (1/2lb)	250g
4 fluid oz (1/2 cup)	125ml	12oz (3/4lb)	375g
8 fluid oz (1 cup)	250ml	16oz (1lb)	500g
1 pint (20 fluid oz/2½ cups)	625ml	24oz (1½lb)	750g
1 pint (US & Canada) (16 fluid oz)	500ml	32oz (2lb)	1kg

Cake Tins

6 inch - 15 cm   Loaf Tin: 9" x 5" - 23 x 12 cm
7 inch - 18 cm   Bar Tin: 10" x 3" - 25 x 8 cm
9 inch - 23 cm   Lamington: 11" x 7" - 28 x 18 cm

Oven Temperature Guide

	Electric		Gas		
	°C	°F	°C	°F	Mark
Cool	110	225	100	200	1/4
Very Slow	120	250	120	250	1/2
Slow	150	300	150	300	1 - 2
Moderately Slow	170	340	160	325	3
Moderate	200	400	180	350	4
Moderately Hot	220	425	190	375	5 - 6
Hot	230	450	200	400	6 - 7
Very Hot	250	475	230	450	8 - 9

CUP AND SPOON EQUIVALENTS IN OUNCES & GRAMS

INGREDIENT	1/2oz 15g	1oz 30g	2oz 60g	3oz 90g	4oz 125g	5oz 150g	6oz 180g	7oz 210g	8oz 250g
Almonds:									
ground	2T	1/4C	1/2C	3/4C	1-1/4C	1-1/3C	1-2/3C	2C	2-1/4C
Apples, dried	3T	1/2C	1C	1-1/3C	2C	2-1/3C	2-3/4C	3-1/3C	3-3/4C
Apricots:									
chopped	2T	1/4C	1/2C	3/4C	1C	1-1/4C	1-1/2C	1-3/4C	2C
whole	2T	3T	1/2C	2/3C	1C	1-1/4C	1-1/3C	1-1/2C	1-3/4C
Arrowroot	1T	2T	1/3C	1/2C	2/3C	3/4C	1C	1-1/4C	1-1/3C
Baking Pdr	1T	2T	1/3C	1/2C	2/3C	3/4C	1C	1C	1-1/4C
Barley	1T	2T	1/4C	1/2C	2/3C	3/4C	1C	1C	1-1/4C
Bicarb. Soda	1T	2T	1/3C	1/2C	2/3C	3/4C	1C	1C	1-1/4C
Breadcrumbs:									
dry	2T	1/4C	1/2C	3/4C	1C	1-1/4C	1-1/2C	1-3/4C	2C
soft	1/4C	1/2C	1C	1-1/2C	2C	2-1/2C	3C	3-2/3C	4-1/4C
Biscuit Crumbs	2T	1/4C	1/2C	3/4C	1-1/4C	1-1/3C	1-2/3C	2C	2-1/4C
Butter	3t	6t	1/4C	1/3C	1/2C	2/3C	3/4C	1C	1C
Cheese grated:									
nat. cheddar	6t	1/4C	1/2C	3/4C	1C	1-1/4C	1-1/2C	1-3/4C	2C
proc. cheddar	5t	2T	1/3C	2/3C	3/4C	1C	1-1/4C	1-1/2C	1-2/3C
Parmesan and Romano	6t	1/4C	1/2C	3/4C	1C	1-1/3C	1-2/3C	2C	2-1/4C
Cherries glace									
chopped	1T	2T	1/3C	1/2C	3/4C	1C	1C	1-1/3C	1-1/2C
whole	1T	2T	1/3C	1/2C	2/3C	3/4C	1C	1-1/4C	1-3/4C
Cocoa	2T	1/4C	1/2C	3/4C	1-1/4C	1-1/3C	1-2/3C	2C	2-1/4C
Coconut, dried	2T	1/3C	2/3C	1C	1-1/3C	1-2/3C	2C	2-1/3C	2-2/3C
shredded	1/3C	2/3C	1-1/4C	1-3/4C	2-1/2C	3C	3-2/3C	4-1/3C	5C
Cornflour	6t	3T	1/2C	2/3C	1C	1-1/4C	1-1/2C	1-2/3C	2C
Coffee: ground	2T	1/3C	2/3C	1C	1-1/3C	1-2/3C	2C	2-1/3C	2-2/3C
instant	3T	1/2C	1C	1-1/3C	1-3/4C	2-1/4C	2-2/3C	3C	3-1/2C
Cornflakes	1/2C	1C	2C	3C	4-1/4C	5-1/4C	6-1/4C	7-1/3C	8-1/3C
Cream of Tartar	1T	2T	1/3C	1/2C	2/3C	3/4C	1C	1C	1-1/4C
Currants	1T	2T	1/3C	2/3C	3/4C	1C	1-1/4C	1-1/2C	1-2/3C
Custard Powdr.	6t	3T	1/2C	2/3C	1C	1-1/4C	1-1/2C	1-2/3C	2C
Dates, choppd	1T	2T	1/3C	2/3C	3/4C	1C	1-1/4C	1-1/2C	1-2/3C
whole, pitted	1T	2T	1/3C	1/2C	3/4C	1C	1-1/4C	1-1/3C	1-1/2C
Figs, chopped	1T	2T	1/3C	1/2C	3/4C	1C	1C	1-1/3C	1-1/2C
Flour, SR, plain	6t	1/4C	1/2C	3/4C	1C	1-1/4C	1-1/2C	1-3/4C	2C
wholemeal	6t	3T	1/2C	2/3C	1C	1-1/4C	1-1/3C	1-2/3C	1-3/4C
Fruit, mixed	1T	2T	1/3C	1/2C	3/4C	1C	1-1/2C	1-1/3C	1-1/2C
Gelatine	5t	2T	1/3C	1/2C	3/4C	1C	1C	1-1/4C	1-1/2C
Ginger:									
crystalised	1T	2T	1/3C	1/2C	3/4C	1C	1-1/4C	1-1/3C	1-1/2C
ground	6t	1/3C	1/2C	3/4C	1-1/4C	1-1/2C	1-3/4C	2C	2-1/4C
in syrup	1T	2T	1/3C	1/2C	2/3C	3/4C	1C	1C	1-1/4C
Glucose, liquid	2t	1T	2T	1/4C	1/3C	1/2C	1/2C	2/3C	2/3C
Golden Syrup	2t	1T	2T	1/4C	1/3C	1/2C	1/2C	2/3C	2/3C
Haricot Beans	1T	2T	1/3C	1/2C	2/3C	3/4C	1C	1C	1-1/4C

t = teaspoonful   T = tablespoonful   C = cupful

CUP AND SPOON EQUIVALENTS IN OUNCES & GRAMS

INGREDIENT	1/2oz 15g	1oz 30g	2oz 60g	3oz 90g	4oz 125g	5oz 150g	6oz 180g	7oz 210g	8oz 250g
Honey	2t	1T	2T	1/4C	1/3C	1/2C	1/2C	2/3C	2/3C
Jam	2t	1T	2T	1/4C	1/3C	1/2C	1/2C	2/3C	3/4C
Lentils	1T	2T	1/3C	1/2C	2/3C	3/4C	1C	1C	1-1/4C
Macaroni	1T	2T	1/3C	1/2C	2/3C	3/4C	1C	1-1/4C	1-1/2C	1-2/3C
Milk Powder:									
full cream	2T	1/4C	1/2C	3/4C	1-1/4C	1-1/3C	1-2/3C	2C	2-1/4
non fat	2T	1/3C	3/4C	1-1/4C	1-1/2C	2C	2-1/3C	2-3/4C	3-1/4C
Nutmeg	6t	3T	1/2C	2/3C	3/4C	1C	1-1/4C	1-1/2C	1-2/3C
Nuts, chop'd	6t	1/4C	1/2C	3/4C	1C	1-1/4C	1-1/2C	1-3/4C	2C
Oatmeal	1T	2T	1/2C	2/3C	3/4C	1C	1-1/4C	1-1/2C	1-2/3C
Olives whole	1T	2T	1/3C	2/3C	3/4C	1C	1-1/4C	1-1/2C	1-2/3C
sliced	1T	2T	1/3C	2/3C	3/4C	1C	1-1/4C	1-1/2C	1-2/3C
Pasta, short	1T	2T	1/3C	2/3C	3/4C	1C	1-1/4C	1-1/2C	1-2/3C
Peaches:									
dried whole	1T	2T	1/3C	2/3C	3/4C	1C	1-1/4C	1-1/2C	1-2/3C
chopped	6t	1/4C	1/2C	3/4C	1C	1-1/4C	1-1/2C	1-3/4C	2C
Peanuts:									
shelled raw	1T	2T	1/3C	1/2C	3/4C	1C	1-1/4C	1-1/3C	1-1/2C
roasted	1T	2T	1/3C	2/3C	3/4C	1C	1-1/4C	1-1/2C	1-2/3C
Peanut Butter	3t	6t	3T	1/3C	1/2C	1/2C	2/3C	3/4C	1C
Peas, split	1T	2T	1/3C	1/2C	2/3C	3/4C	1C	1C	1-1/4C
Peel, mixed	1T	2T	1/3C	1/2C	3/4C	1C	1C	1-1/4C	1-1/2C
Potato: flakes	1/4C	1/2C	1C	1-1/3C	2C	2-1/3C	2-3/4C	3-1/3C	3-3/4C
powdered	1T	2T	1/4C	1/3C	1/2C	2/3C	3/4C	1C	1-1/4C
Prunes:									
chopped	1T	2T	1/3C	1/2C	2/3C	3/4C	1C	1-1/4C	1-1/3C
whole pitted	1T	2T	1/3C	1/2C	2/3C	3/4C	1C	1C	1-1/4C
Raisins	2T	1/4C	1/3C	1/2C	3/4C	1C	1C	1-1/3C	1-1/2C
Rice raw: long	1T	2T	1/3C	1/2C	3/4C	1C	1-1/4C	1-1/3C	1-1/2C
short grain	1T	2T	1/4C	1/2C	2/3C	3/4C	1C	1C	1-1/4C
Rice bubbles	2/3C	1-1/4C	2-1/4C	3-2/3C	5C	6-1/4C	7-1/2C	8-3/4C	10C
Rolled Oats	2T	1/3C	2/3C	1C	1-1/3C	1-3/4C	2C	2-1/2C	2-3/4C
Sago	2T	1/4C	1/3C	1/2C	3/4C	1C	1C	1-1/4C	1-1/2C
Salt	3t	6t	1/4C	1/3C	1/2C	2/3C	3/4C	1C	1C
Semolina	1T	2T	1/3C	1/2C	3/4C	1C	1C	1-1/3C	1-1/2C
Spices	6t	3T	1/4C	1/3C	1/2C	1/2C	2/3C	3/4C	1C
Sugar	3t	6t	1/4C	1/3C	1/2C	1/2C	2/3C	3/4C	1C	1C
Sugar castor	3t	5t	1/4C	1/3C	1/2C	1/2C	2/3C	3/4C	1C	1-1/4C
Sugar, icing	1T	2T	1/3C	1/2C	2/3C	3/4C	1C	1-1/4C	1-1/2C
Sugar, brown	1T	2T	1/3C	1/2C	3/4C	1C	1C	1-1/3C	1-1/2C
Sultanas	1T	2T	1/3C	1/2C	3/4C	1C	1C	1-1/4C	1-1/2C
Tapioca	1T	2T	1/3C	1/2C	2/3C	3/4C	1C	1-1/4C	1-1/3C
Treacle	2t	1T	2T	1/4C	1/3C	1/2C	1/2C	2/3C	2/3C
Walnuts:									
chopped	2T	1/4C	1/2C	3/4C	1C	1-1/4C	1-1/2C	1-3/4C	2C
halved	2T	1/3C	2/3C	1C	1-1/4C	1-1/2C	1-3/4C	2-1/4C	2-1/2C
Yeast: dried	6t	3T	1/2C	2/3C	1C	1-1/4C	1-1/3C	1-2/3C	1-3/4C
compressed	3t	6t	3T	1/3C	1/2C	1/2C	2/3C	3/4C	1C

My favourite recipes

Best-selling Recipe Books
from Southern Holdings

The Australian Apple Recipe Book
Includes 148 top recipes, plus orchard photographs and calendar, apple varieties, and historical apples. 8th reprint.

The Australian Convict Recipe Book
Includes 150 practical recipes, plus historical photographs, convict rules & rations, and the unabridged story of Bessie Baldwin.

The Great Australian Pumpkin Recipe Book
Includes 110 pumpkin recipes (including ice cream), plus the Great Pumpkin story and Growing & Caring for Pumpkins.

The Australian Potato Surprise Recipe Book
155 top potato recipes for all occasions; the versatility of this universal food is fully explored.

The Australian Historical Recipe Book
Join John Caire in exploring Australia's most popular recipes over the years, including some introduced from Europe and Asia. Includes historical photographs and the story,"*Living Off the Land.*" Features Bush & Spade recipes, Steamboat cooking, and Homestead recipes, as well as John's own restaurant recipes.

The Australian Huon Valley Recipe Book
Authentic country recipes from the fine food centre of Tasmania. Selected from treasured family recipe collections. Beautiful Huon scenes and the settlement story are included.

The Australian Heritage Recipe Book
A balanced collection of the most popular tried and true family recipes; this is a book to treasure over years to come. Available in June, 1994

Recipe Books, per copy: $6.95 plus $1.60 P.& P.
(Fundraisers, please enquire about our special offer)
ORDER BY MAIL, PHONE OR FAX FROM:
Southern Holdings Pty Ltd P.O. Huonville 7109, Australia.
Phone: (002)664112; Fax: (002)664112. Credit card orders accepted. All orders sent return mail by Australia Post.